In Search of
Parenthood

In Search of Parenthood

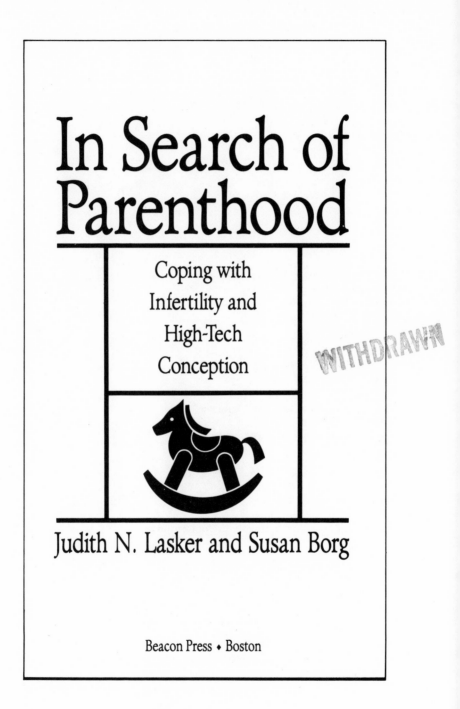

Coping with
Infertility and
High-Tech
Conception

Judith N. Lasker and Susan Borg

Beacon Press ◆ Boston

Beacon Press
25 Beacon Street
Boston, Massachusetts 02108

Beacon Press books
are published under the auspices of
the Unitarian Universalist Association of Congregations.

94 93 92 91 90 89 88 87   8 7 6 5 4 3 2 1

Library of Congress Cataloging-in-Publication Data

Lasker, Judith, 1947–
   In search of parenthood.

   Bibliography: p.
   Includes index.
    1. Human reproduction—Technological innovations—
Psychological aspects.   I. Borg, Susan, 1947–
II. Title.
QP251.L37   1987   362.1'9692   86–47863
ISBN 0–8070–2706–5

Contents

Effects on the Family

Acknowledgments

Without the help of hundreds of people this book would not have been possible. We want each one of them to know that our words of gratitude are deeply felt.

The many women and men who were willing to share their private pain and their experiences with infertility and new technologies are the heart of this book. In addition, the surrogate mothers and sperm and embryo donors whom we interviewed gave us valuable insights into the vital role of the "third parent" in many of these new methods. We have changed people's names and personal descriptions and combined their stories, but we have also tried hard to be true to their words and their feelings.

We are grateful to the professionals who shared their experiences and expertise with us. They gave us insights into the excitement, the frustrations, and the doubts. In many cases, they helped us find people willing to be interviewed about their experiences as donors, surrogate mothers, or clients of fertility programs. We list their names here, the attorneys, nurses, physicians, psychiatrists, psychologists, researchers, and social workers, with a sincere thank you: Howard Adelman, Ph.D., Linda Applegarth, Ed.D., Kenneth J. Borg, Esq., Annette Brodsky, Ph.D., John Buster, M.D., Diane Clapp, R.N., Alan DeCherney, M.D., Anne Marie DeLise, R.N., Robert Echenberg, M.D., Jairo Garcia, M.D., Gale Golden, M.S.W., Dorothy Greenfield, M.S.W., Hilary Hanafin, Ph.D., Ellen Herrenkohl, Ph.D., Gary Hodgen, Ph.D., James Holman, M.D., Pat Humphries, R.N., Elaine Ishita, R.N., Noel Keane, Esq., Ekkehard Kemmann, M.D., Andrea Koch,

Ph.D., Gregory Lang, M.D., Linda Lynch, Dorie McArthur, Ph.D., Hugh Melnick, M.D., Dorothy Mitchell, R.N., Fanny Nero, R.N., Samuel Pasquale, M.D., Zev Rosenwaks, M.D., Barbara Katz Rothman, Ph.D., Burton Satzberg, Esq., Marion Sokolik, M.S.W., James Twerdahl.

Our thanks to the RESOLVE organization, both its national and many local chapters, which published our request for people to interview and provided us with valuable information and connections.

Many friends and colleagues read and commented on selected chapters. We thank the following people for the time and thought they gave to making the writing as clear, complete, and accurate as possible: Diane Clapp, Amy Miller Cohen, Robert Cohen, Jackie DiGerlando, Ann Ehrenkrantz, Joel Ehrenkrantz, Katie Griffiths, Ellen Herrenkohl, Mary Ann Hughes, Susan Lippa, Rosemary Merrill, Debby Nolan, Joan Odes, Carole Reese, Carol Selman, Jane Stein, Kandi Stinson, Susan Turkel, and Sheryl Weinstein. Barbara Katz Rothman has been a valuable colleague and friend; she contributed in many ways to this book and also made extensive comments on the final draft.

A number of Lehigh University students played important roles in the research for this book, both searching out the literature and assisting with the data from two surveys we conducted. Many thanks to Deborah Fleischer, Mary Ann Hughes, Ken Litwin, Mary Loder, Alice Mesaros, Brenda Panichi, and Linda Wimpfheimer.

Annamae Van Doren, Jeanne Chinnock, and Carol Wranovic did an excellent job of transcribing the tapes of interviews, and Judy Specht provided a great deal of clerical support. Tom, Suzanne, and especially Sandy Kelly made the typing, multiple revisions, and completion of the manuscript a family project. We thank them for the many lost weekends and for being available and helpful at all times.

This project has been expensive, including travel to infertility programs, typing and transcribing, telephone calls, equipment and supplies, and research assistance costs. We are grateful to Lehigh University for providing the financial resources needed through several sources: the Class of 1961 Professorship, the Unsponsored Research Fund, the Technology Studies Resource Center, and the Biomedical Research Support Grant. The Department of Social Relations and the Center for Social Research at

Lehigh have also provided important moral support and material assistance for the completion of this work.

Since we live in different states, we have had to find a midway point in which to meet and work. Parts of this book were written in various diners and public libraries in western New Jersey. A special note of thanks to the wonderful librarians in Washington, New Jersey, who made us feel so much at home in our search for a place to work.

Our thanks to Joanne Wyckoff, our editor, for her valuable help with the manuscript and her advice and support throughout the creation of the book. We have been pleased to be associated with Joanne Wyckoff and her colleagues at Beacon Press, where high standards are matched with humanist ideals. We thank Kathryn Gohl for her meticulous and thoughtful editing.

Our families have contributed tremendously to this book. A special thanks to Alan Oransky for comments and suggestions and to Marcia Eskin for her help and support.

Our parents, as always, have taught, guided, and encouraged us. We so much appreciate their advice and their pride. Ruth and Manny Oransky have been very supportive, and Ruth's generous assistance with the children has been indispensable. Miriam and Arnold Lasker, in addition to sending valuable articles regularly, read almost every draft of every chapter. They gave enormously of their time, energy, and expertise to help us organize and present our thoughts clearly. Their wisdom has marked almost every page.

Our husbands, Barry Siegel and Andy Borg, read and commented on many portions of the book. More important, they patiently endured the constant demands on them created by our frequent absences from home over several years of work. We thank them for their love and understanding.

Our daughters, Shira, Laura, Margo, and Ariella, have done more than anyone else to help us appreciate the "search for parenthood." Their lives have been a miracle for us. We thank them for their inspiration and for the joy they have given us.

Introduction

Many people have asked us how we came to write this book together. They wondered why two women, one a sociologist living in Pennsylvania and the other an architect in New Jersey, drove hundreds of miles each week to write about infertility.

We met over thirty years ago, in Mrs. Cosgrove's kindergarten class. We grew up together, around the corner from each other, sharing the play and dreams of childhood. In all of those years spent in each other's homes and on the phone together, we rarely talked about having children. We just assumed that one day, when the time was right, we would become mothers.

Years later we both discovered, tragically, how false that assumption had been. Within a horrible period of six months, we each watched our firstborn baby die. From our experiences we learned that pregnancy does not always occur easily and that healthy babies should not be taken for granted. We relied on each other for comfort and for support in our grief. Out of that sharing came *When Pregnancy Fails: Families Coping With Miscarriage, Stillbirth, and Infant Death,* a book we wrote about the experience of loss in pregnancy.[1]

We have spoken about miscarriage and infant loss to many groups in the past few years. Because of our writing and speaking, we have met thousands of men and women who also grieve for the babies they have lost. Each one of them reminds us that creating a healthy baby is an intricate, miraculous process that goes wrong far too often.

Many of the people we have met are struggling with infertility as well. Their stories of grief for the children they cannot have touched us deeply. We felt their pain and frustration even more strongly because of personal encounters with infertility. We realized that there is almost no understanding from others for this kind of loss. From our awareness of the enormous impact of infertility and the many changes occurring in its treatment came the desire to write *In Search of Parenthood*.

Most people like us who have struggled to become parents started out thinking they had some control over their lives. We all grew up with the revolutionary idea of reproductive choice. With more effective birth control and legalized abortion we could plan when (or if) we wanted to have children. We have arrived painfully at the realization that we really have little control. The idea of "reproductive freedom" is a cruel reminder of what we thought we were entitled to and discovered we have lost.

Becoming a parent seems as though it should be easier than ever before. There is much greater knowledge about reproduction and many new treatments for infertility. Yet the most advanced medical technologies and the best efforts of both prospective parents and health professionals cannot guarantee success. Millions of Americans are now caught up in a desperate search to have a baby.

Why do so many people have trouble conceiving? Infections, venereal diseases, and environmental toxins are all important factors affecting the fertility of both men and women. As couples wait longer to begin having children, there is more time to be exposed to these hazards. In addition, medical care itself has caused some infertility. Some birth control measures, especially the Dalkon Shield IUD have fostered infections that destroyed women's reproductive organs. DES, a hormone given to pregnant women several decades ago, caused infertility in many of their children years later. Even cesarean sections might increase the chance of problems because of infections and scarring that may result from surgery.[2]

The National Center for Health Statistics estimates from a national survey that more than one in every five couples in the United States, or over 12 million people, have difficulty conceiving or carrying a child. This number includes the many people who have been sterilized for noncontraceptive reasons. Of course, not everyone whose fertility is impaired wants to have a child or additional children. However, more than half of the women in couples with fertility problems said that they would like a child if it were possible. Adoption has become increasingly difficult or unavailable. As a result, the demand for infertility services has grown enormously. This demand is particularly strong among the growing numbers of middle- and upper-middle-class educated people in their thirties who are infertile. They are people with resources but, because of their age, not much time to wait. Medical, legal, and scientific professionals have rushed in to respond to this situation. The result has been that the number of infertility-related programs has multiplied in the last few years.[3]

These programs promise exciting new alternatives that may help fulfill the dreams of people who want so much to be parents. But they also carry with them high emotional and financial costs. In this book, we examine the new technologies—the hope they offer as well as the difficult dilemmas and personal challenges they present.

The methods we look at are artificial insemination with sperm from the husband (AIH) or from a donor (AID), in vitro (better known as test-tube) fertilization (IVF), surrogate motherhood, and ovum transfer (OT) from a donor woman. Although there are many possible treatments for infertility, these are the most publicized and the most controversial. Variations on each method are being developed all the time, and new terms such as GIFT (gamete intrafallopian transfer) have appeared. While the alternatives are very different from each other, the attention they have received, in contrast to other infertility treatments, is largely due to their being methods of conceiving a child without sexual intercourse.

Much of the research on which the methods are based was originally intended to help cattle breeders and has been going on for decades. Only in the last few years have these methods begun to be widely available for solving problems of human infertility. As treatments are perfected and the concern about infertility continues to rise, the people trying these methods will number in the hundreds of thousands worldwide.

Infertile people now make up the greatest portion of those who are interested in the alternatives. Other situations might also lead people to consider them. One member of a couple might carry a genetic trait he or she does not want to risk passing on to a child. There are women for whom pregnancy may be dangerous. Single heterosexual or gay men and women who want to become parents without sexual involvement are increasingly using AID and surrogate programs. Although in this book we refer primarily to infertile couples, we intend our comments to apply to anyone who has difficulty conceiving or carrying a healthy baby.

Many critics are concerned that surrogate mothers will be hired for convenience by women who simply do not wish to be pregnant, or that IVF and AID will be used to create superior children with selected genetic traits. These are very real worries, and the direction of research raises troubling questions for the future. But our concern here is for the people who would like nothing better than to conceive the "old-fashioned" way. For them, the alternatives are not a convenience or an adventure. They are a last resort.

A great deal has already been written about these alternatives. Important books and articles examine carefully the legal, ethical, or political problems raised by the new technologies. Some authors extol the wonders of the new discoveries and explain the technical aspects in detail. Others condemn them as ethically questionable, religiously unacceptable, or socially dangerous.[4]

Our purpose is a different one. We examine the impact of these methods on the many people whose lives they touch—the hopeful parents and their families, the donors and surrogate mothers, the professionals, and of course the children. We look at the personal side, the emotional impact of the technology. The technical details are changing extraordinarily fast, as almost every week brings publicity about new developments. Legal considerations are also undergoing some changes. But the feelings and concerns of the people involved, which is the focus of this book, remain basically the same.

These methods are bringing enormous benefits to many people, but they also present many emotional risks and potential physical dangers. No one knows for sure what long-term effects these new medical procedures may have on the mothers and fathers or on the children.

People already feeling vulnerable because they have not been able to have children now face unprecedented dilemmas and decisions. How much are they willing to go through to try to have a child? Can they find the right resources? Can they afford it? Should they tell anyone? Can they take the added stress and physical risk? How do they feel about being part of an experiment, doing something others may condemn? How should they relate to the person who provided the semen or the egg or who carried the baby for them?

As we consider these questions, we address the differences in the ways men and women tend to respond to them. These differences often create difficult times for couples already under great stress. They may disagree on how important it is to have a biological child rather than adopt, or on how much to share the news of what they are doing with friends, or on what they will later tell the child. The responses to these issues are often very different depending on whether it is the man or the woman who has been identified as infertile.

The new methods give even greater power to scientists and physicians. Now they not only assist couples to conceive on their own; they actually "perform" the conception themselves in their offices or laboratories. They are storing the beginnings of life in "banks" and, in many cases, turning their practices into commercial ventures. We discuss the implications of this increasing medical control over life. How does it affect the people who are now turning to these professionals, looking for emotional support as well as medical expertise? And what about the much greater number who cannot afford even to consider the possibilities? How will this medical control affect all of us in the future?

The public knows little about the donors who are more and more involved in these efforts to conceive. We compare the motivations and experiences of the anonymous sperm donors to those of the women who contract to conceive and carry a baby for someone else. Is it really so easy for any of them?

The new technologies have challenged us to reconsider what we mean by a parent or by a family. For instance, these technologies are giving single people, both homosexual and heterosexual, greater options for parenthood. Some parents are including donors as part of their families. The possibilities for control over conception raise numerous questions for society, about social relationships, about eugenics and sex selection, and about what kind of children we want and how we want to have them.[5]

In the heated debates that have emerged around these new alternatives, we find it impossible to join those who take positions that are clearly for or against. The more we study the experiences of people trying these methods, the more we feel torn between the two sides of this debate.

Both of us have known the anguish of not having the baby we wanted so much. Now that we are mothers, with living children who are so central to our lives, we cannot imagine anyone taking away our chance of having them. We have also seen the incredible joy of people who have finally had babies after all else failed. Because of these experiences, we feel reluctant to see any option eliminated that would help people who want to become parents.

There is another side to this situation though. We worry a lot about the abuses likely to result from commercializing conception. We fear the possibilities of exploitation of surrogates and of profiteering at the expense of infertile people. We have little confidence, after seeing past abuses, that scientific discoveries in the field of reproduction will be used only to help people. We have also seen people pressured into trying an expensive and stressful method simply because it was there, only to meet with renewed devastation from one more failure. We have learned of patients deceived about the likelihood of success and led on by physicians with little experience.

In spite of what we have learned, we find ourselves sometimes recommending one or another of these alternatives. We understand the desperate need of our friends to become parents. Yet we also warn them that this is not easy, that they need to know exactly what they are getting into.

◆　◆　◆　◆　◆

Our review of the literature in medicine, sociology, psychology, law, and ethics has given us some information about the issues we considered important in writing this book. But we knew the best insights would come from talking with people who had experienced the various methods. We wondered at first, since these methods were quite new, if we could find men and women who would share their stories with us.

It was easier to find people than we had expected because so many lives are affected by infertility. Some people were referred to us by physicians and staff members of IVF and surrogate programs; others were found through personal contacts. The largest number were people who responded to our requests for assistance in both national and local newsletters of RESOLVE, a support organization for infertile people.

To a large extent, then, our sample consists of volunteers and does not represent all people who are infertile or who try alternative methods of conception. This study should be considered exploratory, one that has attempted to uncover the important personal issues raised by the new alternatives.

Between 1984 and 1986 we interviewed people from all over the country, in person and by phone, and collected questionnaires through the mail. Many people represented here have tried one or more of the alternatives; some have considered them and decided not to go on. Some have had successful pregnancies, others have not and are still trying to conceive. Many have adopted children.

We visited programs throughout the country, interviewing physicians, nurses, lawyers, and therapists. We wrote to all the in vitro fertilization centers, requesting information about the programs and their success rates. We also interviewed the donors— surrogate mothers and sperm and embryo donors. Altogether over two hundred people have directly contributed their experiences to this book.

We also wanted to find out more about the attitudes of people not directly affected by infertility. We surveyed 165 students at two colleges in Pennsylvania to obtain their views on the new alternatives. In addition, we investigated existing polls and national surveys to learn the opinions of the general public and the ways they have changed over time.

We hope that, by reading this book, people who are considering these methods will have a clearer picture of what they are likely to face. Those who have already begun, or finished, trying an alternative should recognize that their experiences and emotions are shared by many others. Also, we want professionals to understand their clients' experiences so that services might better meet the clients' needs. And we hope the general public will gain a more complete idea of what these significant changes mean.

◆　◆　◆　◆　◆

Since our personal tragedies we have, between us, given birth to three healthy babies and have adopted an infant. We have been through the travails of fertility treatment, the anxieties of prenatal testing, and the struggle for successful birth uncomplicated by excessive intervention. We feel like survivors, attuned to the fragility of birth and life by our personal experiences.

We look at our kindergarten class pictures now and see two curly-haired smiling girls for whom the world was so simple. We would never have believed then, nor even understood, the joys and tragedies of childbirth that would join our lives and our work so many years later.

The Trauma of Infertility

1
The Drive to Have Children

We'll sell the car, the house even, if it comes to it. . . . There was nothing I wouldn't give up if it meant we could have a child.[1]

Over and over we have heard such words of desperation, of willingness to endure any pain or expense, even to risk one's life, all in order to have a child. The search for parenthood by infertile people has been compared to a terminal cancer victim's quest for a cure. But infertility, though painful, is not life threatening. Why are people so driven in their efforts?

Personal and Social Pressures

Gail is a thirty-four-year-old woman who has been through eight cycles of AIH (artificial insemination with her husband's sperm) and four attempts at IVF (test-tube fertilization) in the last five years, all without success. Gail is a calm, good-natured person, but she describes herself as "driven" to keep trying to get pregnant:

> It's worth it all to know you've done everything that you can do. I don't want to always be wondering if we should have pushed a little harder or tried something else. At least I know my inability to conceive is not from lack of trying.

What is it about conceiving and bearing children that is so crucial to infertile people like Gail, that makes them willing to try almost anything? Some scientists, agreeing with Harvard sociobiologist Edward O. Wilson's theories, claim that people's desire to reproduce is innate, perhaps even programmed into their genes. Although there may be a biological component to wanting to bear children, no one has yet been able to prove or measure it. On the contrary, a great deal of evidence shows that social and psychological pressures to have children are at least as powerful, if not more so, than the biological pressures.[2]

Gail's desire for children is like that of many other people. She talks about feelings of emptiness, the sense that her family is not yet complete. She and her husband Bill have been married for nine years, and they are eager to share their love with children. They yearn for the pleasure of cuddling babies and playing with them as they grow. They want to pass on their values, to see themselves as living on in the future through the lives of their children.

Gail and Bill's own internal drive to be parents is strongly reinforced by external pressures. They believe they have made their own choice to have children, but it is obvious that this choice would be greatly approved by others. Gail described the pressures from her family and friends:

> When I was little, my parents talked a lot about what it would be like when I grew up and became a mother. "Growing up" and "becoming a mother" seemed like the same thing. After I got married, the comments started coming in from my friends as well as my parents—"Well, when are you going to have a family?" they kept asking us. They were all having kids, and we felt very left out. I'm sure this all had an impact on our wish for children.
>
> It isn't just my relatives and friends. I think it's in the air, almost like an epidemic. Everywhere I go there are pregnant women and babies, in the stores, on TV, just walking along the street. It makes you feel abnormal not to be pushing a stroller or buying the newest kind of diaper.

The pressures to have children go beyond comments from others and commercials on television. They are deeply imbedded in the culture, supported by powerful social norms.

Every culture has its ideal image of what a man and a woman should be like, and for the woman, the cultural ideal is almost always focused on motherhood. People who do not have children are generally considered selfish and maladjusted, a harsh judgment from society.[3]

The influence of social pressures becomes most obvious when a shift in fertility trends occurs. In the United States, for example, there have been dramatic changes over the last few decades in the number of children per family. In the aftermath of World War II, women were encouraged to have large families, and the birth rate rose sharply. Then, in the late 1960s and early 1970s, fertility dropped steadily. Childlessness became more acceptable, and small families were preferred. Now, in the 1980s, the pressures seem to have gone in the opposite direction once again. Children of the postwar baby boom are now having children, and the result is a rise in the number of babies being born and a great deal of public attention to pregnancy and childbirth.[4]

These changes are responses to the economic and political climate of the time, not simply the accumulation of millions of individual decisions. We all like to think that such important decisions as whether or not to have children and how many to have are made by ourselves, independently. Yet our behavior, consciously or unconsciously, is often strongly influenced by prevailing social trends.

The pressures to have children affect not only married couples. A growing number of single women are turning to technological means of conception because of their desire to have children.[5]

The demands of others also affect those who already have one child. If having no children is selfish, having one and denying him or her the chance to have siblings is said to be cruel. "Only children" are stereotyped as spoiled and maladjusted, despite considerable evidence to the contrary. In fact, a study by sociologist Nancy Russo found that the plan to have one child is almost as unpopular among Americans as the goal of having none. This attitude makes the frequent situation of secondary infertility even more difficult for people who are trying so hard to have another child.[6]

Why should it be necessary to pressure people to have children? If the notion were true that children bring the ultimate fulfillment (especially for women), then no one would need encouragement. But having children can be a very risky business.

National surveys all agree that couples without children are happier with their marriages than those who do have children.

Satisfaction with marriage starts to drop shortly after the first child arrives, increasing again only after the last child leaves home.[7]

Women, paradoxically, suffer the most from having children. Mothers are more likely to be depressed than nonmothers. And women who, without children, are equal to their husbands in almost every way in their marriage, quickly discover that the arrival of a child sharply reduces their power in marital decision making. Even women who continue working outside of the home lose power as they become defined as primary caretaker and homemaker.[8]

Of course there is another very different reality—that children can be wonderful, that parenting can be the most satisfying experience in one's life. Having children is neither pure heaven nor total hell but some combination of both. The vast majority of people keep their eyes fixed on the positive, the beautiful, and take the risk. They count on the miracle of new life and the love that children bring. They cannot imagine going through life without them.

It is understandable why many people like Gail who cannot have children are so desperate. They have failed to fulfill their own desires, their expectations of what their lives would be like. They have also failed to fulfill the powerful mandate of society, but not by any choice of their own. And they feel the stigma attached to anyone who deviates from the most central norms of society. It is no wonder some people are willing to undergo enormous stress and risk to become parents.[9]

Why Not Adopt?

If the goal were primarily to be parents, it should not matter so much where the children come from. Gail told us she is asked by some of her friends, "Why not just adopt?"

> They don't seem to understand why, for me, adoption is still a last resort. It just is not the same as having a biological child.

The social norm is not only to be a parent; it is to be a biological parent. We are urged to create new life, to perpetuate the species.

Most of the people who responded to our questionnaires and interviews indicated that they had indeed considered adoption or were already on a waiting list. The fact remains, however, that almost all of them (including some who had already adopted one child) were still pursuing other alternatives. Why don't they give up on trying to conceive, especially after repeated failures? Why do they reject adoption or turn to it only as a last resort?

Adoption is risky and difficult. Waiting lists for healthy infants are long. The costs are exorbitant. Adoption agency caseworkers ask many personal questions, make judgments, and have excessive control over one's life. Some people simply are not eligible. These are the reasons people gave us for not wanting to pursue adoption.

But infertility procedures are often described in exactly the same terms. Programs are impersonal; waiting for results is unbearable. Failure rates are high, and costs are prohibitive for many. Even so, most people prefer to try infertility treatments, with all their problems, rather than face the difficulties of adoption. There is one very basic reason for this choice: most people want a biological child.

All those who filled out our questionnaire and said they had rejected adoption as an alternative cited the desire for a biological child as the reason. Those who try the reproductive alternatives go through all of the trouble and stress not only to be parents, but to create their "own" children.[10]

Becoming parents is very closely tied, in the minds of many, to the proper functioning of their bodies. A man sees a biological child as proof of his virility. For a woman, a biological child means being able to experience pregnancy, birth, and breast-feeding. For both, the inability to produce a child is a threat to their sexual identity.

For many people, genes are the key issue. As Bill said:

Gail is really smart and pretty, and I feel good about myself. It would be neat to see our qualities passed on to a child. And we worry about how healthy or intelligent an adopted child would be. At least with our own, we think we'd have a pretty good idea of what we'd be getting.

Some people worry about the effects of adoption on children, especially foreign-born or biracial children. Having "one's own" seems so much less complicated. It is certainly more acceptable to the world around us.

A child is the most visible demonstration of a couple's love for each other, a miraculous creation that comes out of the intimate union of two people. One woman expressed her regret at losing this possibility:

> The hardest part of all of this has been dealing with the idea of our lovemaking not producing a little part of ourselves, melted together. I still miss my husband's smile or his eyes in our adopted son, although I love him dearly.

Men usually appear to be the driving force behind the preference for a biological child. Many women told us they would be happy to adopt, but that their husbands wanted a genetic connection. The men agreed. Why the difference?

Genes are the biggest contribution men make to the creation of a child. They cannot carry, birth, or nurse a baby. In addition, they are rarely the major care-giver. Women can "mother" in many ways. Many men, especially those who have not yet experienced the daily caring and loving that fathering can entail, focus on the biological connection.

Gail explained her husband's reluctance to adopt:

> Bill thought he would feel more comfortable with a child that was ours biologically. He says he just couldn't accept an adopted child as his own.

Men may also be more concerned with carrying on the family name and heritage. One man who learned he was infertile explained:

> The hardest part was telling my father. I felt like I had failed him. I had broken the chain, the idea of continuity from the past to the future which still seems so important in some primitive part of ourselves.

When adoption was easier, it may have been a more acceptable solution. In any case, it was often the only alternative to childlessness. Today, the situation is dramatically different. People keep trying to have biological children not only because they want them and not only because of social pressures, but also because infertility specialists are promising new alternatives. It has become increasingly difficult for infertile people to say no to this new set of pressures.

The Pressure to Keep Trying

An individual's desire to keep trying to have a baby is powerfully reinforced from the outside—from media accounts of miracle babies, from acquaintances who have been successful, and from friends who encourage one to try a new method they have heard about. One woman told us she felt overly pressured by optimistic news reports:

If I see one more article or book that says. "You *can* have a baby," or "New hope for childless couples," I think I'll scream. Sure it's good for the public to know, but the message seems to be that if you just try hard enough or go to the right doctor you're sure to get pregnant. I wish it were so easy!

The most direct pressure, and the hardest for many to resist, comes from physicians. Almost everyone we surveyed who attempted conception through AIH or AID (artificial insemination with a donor's sperm) cited a doctor's recommendation as the reason. The choice of IVF (in vitro fertilization) was explained as "our last hope," "our only choice," a message that is strongly reinforced by the medical community.

A staff member of an IVF program described the pressure to try alternatives:

More and more it has become a matter of "all roads lead to in vitro." More and more physicians around the country are saying to couples, "Well there's always IVF."

People who do decide to try a new method are usually very persistent, very driven to succeed.[11] They are people, like Gail, who feel compelled to keep going:

For someone who doesn't gamble and hates the idea of getting on a roller coaster, it was quite an effort to decide to try IVF. But at the same time, I found the idea of quitting most frightening. It was as if all the tests, operations and medication through the years would have been for nothing. I just could not face the idea of failure.

Gail is accurate in describing her decision as a gamble, a high-risk venture into the unknown. Gamblers make pacts with themselves (pacts that are often broken) about how much longer they will try to win or how much more money they will spend on each game. Infertile people do the same. They often "hedge their bets" by getting onto adoption lists while trying to conceive. They promise themselves that they will try just "one more time," or "one more year," or until the money runs out.

Every new technique creates new options and new pressures, added possibilities, increased risks. It is hard to decide whether it is worth all of the risks one has to take to pursue another alternative. Is it worth the problems of having a child who is biologically related to only one parent? Is it worth the money? Is it worth the personal stress and physical pain? And most of all, is it worth taking the risk of failing once again?

Many people, despite all of the pressures, eventually decide they have had enough. It is not worth it to them to keep trying, to keep hurting and hoping. They discover that their lives can be fulfilling in ways other than parenting, or that adopted children bring them every joy they had hoped for.

Others decide it is worth the risks, the trouble, the stresses of the treatment. Their commitment to having a biological child compels them to go on, overshadowing other goals. Not being able to have children makes them so unhappy that some are willing to try anything that might help. Theirs is a grief that is often overwhelming, a sense of loss that only success, it seems, can erase.

2
Feelings of Grief

*Once again pregnancy has eluded us. I awake with
moderate cramps and lower back pain. No flow.
Resisting the urge to take Motrin since maybe this is a
false alarm and I might really be pregnant, I endure
several hours of increasingly more severe pain. Finally,
the blood comes. Right on time, my period has started.
And so begins another cycle, a pattern which has
repeated itself again and again over the past 2½ years.*

*As I have done a countless number of times in the
past two weeks, I run to look at my chart. My cervix
was right, my cervical mucus was right, my basal body
temperature was right, and our timing of intercourse
was right. What more could we have done? Clearly,
infertility listens not to fact or reason. It must have
greater weapons in its arsenal.*

*I picture endometriosis down there looking smug and
very certain that it will continue to defeat our every
attempt at pregnancy. And there are my diseased tubes
and ovaries, weak and powerless against this enemy, that
thus far has not been beaten by Danazol or major
surgery.*

*Hope and courage and optimism line up facing despair
and hopelessness and depression, prepared to do battle.
Maybe this cycle pregnancy will be the victor;
endometriosis and infertility, the losers.*

Probably not. [1]

The image of fighting against an unseen enemy captures the feelings of many who struggle with infertility. They feel as if they have been struck by a natural disaster, an unexpected and uncontrollable devastation of their lives. Infertile people grieve with the same emotions as those who grieve for the death of a loved one.

Yet this is a different kind of grief. A death has finality to it, but infertility can go on indefinitely. It is like having a chronic illness; there is the continuing reminder of loss coupled with continued hope for a cure. Each month there is a new hope, the fantasy of being pregnant, the conviction that *this* time it just has to work. Then, once again, the crushing evidence of failure. One woman who wrote an article in the *RESOLVE Newsletter* described it this way:

> Being infertile has been compared to having a loved one missing in action; I hope and grieve simultaneously, a delicate tension.[2]

A death is not only final; it is also a public event, a rallying point for family and friends to offer sympathy and help. Infertility, in contrast, is a very private trauma, unrecognized, and misunderstood by others. Deaths are marked by ceremony and gravestones. Other life crises also have their rituals. But the loss each month of the possibility of a desperately wanted child goes unnoticed, marked only by the purchase of more sanitary napkins. As one woman told us:

> A lot of people don't understand that infertility is very much like having a child die. You grieve for the baby who wasn't conceived this month, and for all the babies you'll never have.

The devastation brought by infertility is hardly a new phenomenon. The Bible, for example, contains a number of stories about women who could not bear children. The book of Samuel opens with one such story, about Hannah. Her grief, like that of so many people, was also misunderstood.

Hannah's husband Elkanah, who loved her very much, could not understand why she was so upset, asking if he was not good enough for her: "Hannah, why do you weep? And why do you not eat? And why is your heart sad? Am I not more to you than ten sons?"

Elkanah's other wife Peninah had children, and she taunted Hannah constantly. Even Eli, the priest in the temple where Hannah went to pray for a child, scorned her. He took her obvious distress to be a sign of drunkenness, until Hannah explained that she was "a woman sorely troubled," filled with "great anxiety and vexation" (1 Sam. 1).

The Grief Process

The grief Hannah felt is a normal response to loss. It is hard to imagine how so much pain and bitterness can be normal and even necessary for coping. But grief has been aptly described to us by a social worker as a circle of fire around a bereaved person. One must walk through and be burned in order to get to the outside, or else stay trapped inside forever. The "burns" of grief wound us in many ways that are common to almost all losses. They are the now widely recognized reactions of shock, denial, anger, guilt, depression, and resolution.[3]

Most couples are *shocked* when they find out they have infertility or genetic problems. They had thought they were largely in control of their future, that surely having children would be part of the natural progression of their lives. They are stunned, disbelieving, when it turns out otherwise. Feeling vulnerable, they are frightened to discover how little control they have over what happens to them.

Since infertility is so uncertain, many people find it easy to *deny* it. "This isn't happening to me," they say. Some denial helps a person adjust to an overwhelming situation. Total denial can be destructive, however, if a couple delays seeking help until it is almost too late to do anything. One man told us about his experience:

> My wife and I were trying hard to have a baby. After a year, my wife's physician didn't seem worried; so we didn't even suspect anything could be wrong. After another year, he thought we should have some tests, but I was sure it was just our timing. How could anything be wrong with us?
>
> It took another year to get me to go get my sperm tested, and I went only because of my wife's insistence. I just didn't want to believe anything could be wrong. Now I wish we hadn't wasted all that time.

Sometimes the grief over being infertile goes underground, unacknowledged. This can happen when a diagnosis of male infertility is followed immediately by a successful AID (artificial insemination with donor sperm) or when a baby becomes unexpectedly available for adoption soon after the detection of blocked tubes. But the feelings do not necessarily disappear. They may reemerge without warning later on, still demanding attention.

Men are more likely than women to deny the problem or their feelings. Women, on the other hand, often deny the incredible rage that is part of the grief of infertility. According to studies, women have a harder time showing their *anger* than men. One woman quoted by psychologist Patricia P. Mahlstedt said:

> My husband told me he hated what the past few years had done to me. He said he watched me turn into an angry, bitter, hateful person. It was a long time before I realized how angry I was. I was consumed with anger before I understood what was eating me up inside. Then my problem was finding what to do with my anger—how at least to channel it, if not resolve it.[4]

Anger and frustration can be all-too-constant companions. Anger at insensitive friends or relatives who say "just relax," "go on vacation," or "adopt and then you'll get pregnant." How could so-called friends be so ignorant, so impatient with the depression and preoccupation infertility causes? Some may find that they no longer can stay in contact with these "friends" who fail to understand. They find themselves feeling isolated and lonely. Family parties become too painful, especially as new nieces, nephews, and cousins appear each year.

Friends and relatives are not the only targets of anger. Doctors, nurses, and hospitals are often high on the list. Infertile people feel very vulnerable to the doctors' control over their lives. They are tired of the endless painful procedures they must endure. They are angry at physicians who have no infertility expertise yet assure that they can help. They are angry at the specialists who have no time for them or who are condescending or insensitive.

One man's comment reveals a common sentiment:

> We foolishly believed everything the various doctors told us. We learned the hard way that we had to cut through the

"we know best" garbage to get accurate information. We had to find the person who really knew what he was doing, instead of wasting so much time with inexperienced gynecologists who claimed to be specialists but really were not.

A woman who was going through AIH (artificial insemination with her husband's sperm) reflected one frequent source of anger at physicians:

I know their time is precious. I know I am only one of many patients. But when they can offer me only one block of time and expect that I should rearrange my whole day on one day's notice and then pay dearly for their time, and this happens over and over every 28 days, it is a source of repeated frustration.

The anger may extend to doctors in general, especially if it is suspected that a medical intervention caused the problem to begin with. DES daughters and women whose infertility was destroyed by IUDs are furious that they must turn for help to a medical system they hold responsible for their trauma.

Many infertile people are upset about the cost and time they spend trying to get pregnant. Many give up their jobs to be available for the tests and procedures. Others may have to mortgage their homes to obtain the thousands of dollars needed for many treatments. One woman wrote us to share her feelings:

One thing about being infertile, you'd better have a large income and good insurance because everything you do to diagnose infertility and to achieve a pregnancy is very expensive and not for the average couple. Maybe someone should sell infertility insurance so when you get married and can't have children, it'll pay for treatment or adoption.

After experiencing a loss or tragedy, at some point people ask themselves, "What could I have done to avoid it?" Even if it is an event totally out of their control, they wonder if God or fate is punishing them. *Guilt,* for real or imagined offenses, is inevitable. But the constant search for a cause, the preoccupation with possible faults, can poison one's life.

The media help fuel the guilt. News reports cite the rise in sexually transmitted diseases as causing the increases in infertility problems, and people begin to wonder about their past relationships. The guilt is even greater if one links infertility to a past abortion. In reality, abortions have not been shown to cause infertility, but it is hard to forget them, especially in the current political environment.[5]

Many decisions we've made in our lives may come back to haunt us, even though they may have been the best decisions at the time. The choice of birth control methods or the decision to wait to have children may have increased the likelihood of infertility. How ironic, how tragic that our efforts to control fertility, to control the course of our lives, may have led directly to our loss of the ability to conceive.

Psychiatrists have long claimed that emotional distress or neurosis can cause infertility. According to such theories, relaxation or therapy is all that is needed to achieve a successful pregnancy. This viewpoint only adds to the burden of guilt. Fortunately, it is now possible to identify organic causes for over 90 percent of infertility.[6] Hard medical evidence has made psychological theories much less convincing. Also, more therapists have recognized that distress is usually a result, not a cause, of infertility.

An exact diagnosis can cause renewed guilt and more questions: "How did my tubes get so scarred?" "Why are my sperm so slow?" "What did I do to make this happen?" But a diagnosis is also an answer and the basis for a treatment strategy. A diagnosis can make it easier to accept the situation, to decide what to do next. The fewer than 10 percent of infertile people who find no cause are therefore doubly frustrated. For example, we interviewed a woman who was undergoing AIH for unexplained infertility. She described her feelings:

> As a woman you just expect to have a baby; so you say to yourself, "What did I do wrong, what's happening inside my body that's not right?" I have an image in my mind of Pac Man. Maybe I have these little things like antibodies eating the sperm, chubba, chubba, chubba. You can get really crazy.

The feelings of guilt, anger, and frustration can turn into serious *depression*. Depression is a frequent response to infertility.

> At this time in my life I wanted a house, I wanted a career. I wanted the kids and everything. Instead I feel that there's nothing left in my life. I wind up renting an apartment from

24

my mother, staying home and cleaning and being very domestic. I haven't been able to work for three years because I have to be on call, going back and forth to the hospital, monitoring urines. Sometimes it seems that things will never get better.

It is hard to make decisions when one is feeling depressed. It is hard to muster the energy needed to investigate all the alternatives, to keep going back for more and more procedures. As one woman said:

Sometimes I feel so low, all I want is to lie in bed. I have to drag myself to the doctor. I know if I don't, I'll have no chance at all.

These feelings of grief—shock, denial, anger, guilt, and depression—are common to all kinds of losses. There are other painful emotions that most discussions of grief neglect, but that can affect infertile people very powerfully. They may have a strong sense of *failure*. Their bodies have failed to perform a very basic function, and their sense of themselves as a man or woman is challenged. One woman said:

Intellectually, I know that this doesn't mean I'm a failure as a wife or a woman or that I'm not feminine. But, as many times as you go through this, your emotions take over and you do feel like a total failure.

Infertile people cannot help but feel *jealous* of others who have had no problems in bearing children. Wherever they go, they feel surrounded by babies and pregnant women. Whenever they watch television, pick up a magazine, or read a paper they are reminded that they live in a fertile, unsympathetic world. Some are especially furious at those parents who neglect and abuse their children. One woman told us bitterly:

I can't even control my own damn body. Other women have babies so easily and just take it for granted. They even plan exactly when they want the baby to arrive—those are the ones that drive me crazy.

Jealousy appears even in groups intended to help infertile people. Psychiatrist Miriam Mazor observes:

Women who have had a series of miscarriages are viewed as "more fortunate" by those who have never conceived;

those who ovulate regularly are seen as "more normal" by those who do not. ... Rarely will they tolerate a member with a secondary infertility problem (one who has borne a living child), and they have difficulty in dealing with the issue of what to do about group members who become pregnant, with the initial impulse being to expel the offending member.[7]

Grief with Secondary Infertility and Pregnancy Loss

Becoming pregnant is a major achievement. But for some it may not, unfortunately, end the grief. Many people have one child and then can have no more. Others experience the loss of a baby.

We tend to think of infertility as being the same as childlessness. It is surprising to realize, then, that of all infertile couples, 60 percent already have one or more children.[8] If they have been trying unsuccessfully to conceive for a year or more, they are considered infertile, no matter how many other children they have.

Those who experience secondary infertility are especially shocked, for their experience makes them feel certain they can be successful again. They also feel even more isolated; others tell them to feel grateful for the child or children they already have. Gjerde Dausch, writing in the *RESOLVE Newsletter,* describes how she hid the existence of her son from her RESOLVE friends. Although she very much wanted another child, people trying to have their first did not consider her infertile. Her response:

> Yes, we have a child, but our problems and feelings are the same. Just because we have one child does not mean we can't or don't mourn the loss of the unborn child.

There is a great deal of guilt associated with secondary infertility. Dausch writes:

> I spent a great deal of time reflecting back on my life to see where I had gone wrong to merit only one child. ... My emotional state, I believe, suffered even more as a result of having a child. I could never tell myself that my infertility was an act of fate or something possessed from birth. Since it was so easy the first time, I felt that I must have done something after his birth to cause my infertility. ... I had

had the ability to have children, and I kept looking for what I did to destroy this.[9]

A new trauma may confront those who actually do conceive. Miscarriage and ectopic (tubal) pregnancy are common early in pregnancy, especially for those with fertility problems.[10] Some people will experience a successful first trimester only to face the heartbreaking news of a genetic problem discovered by a prenatal test such as amniocentesis. They will have to decide whether to end the much wanted pregnancy, whether to abort the child whose obvious movements and growth had brought such joy.

As in any other group of pregnant women, some infertile people who finally conceive will experience premature labor, stillbirth, or newborn death. So close to their goal, they feel betrayed and cheated when they have to bear another loss. One woman who conceived after having infertility problems wrote to us about her feelings about the baby's death:

> When I became pregnant, I really thought that we had won the battle, and would somehow be protected from more problems because we had "paid our dues" with infertility.

Ironically, those who experience such tragedies may find themselves isolated in their bereavement. Their infertile friends may tell them, "At least you got pregnant." In IVF programs, a pregnancy—no matter how brief—is counted as a "success." And they may discover what most others who have lost babies have found: the rest of the world does not understand how disastrous these losses are.

Resolution

Resolution should be the last stage of grief. However, without a recognized loss, with no obvious end to the struggle, with little support from others, resolution is especially hard to achieve.

Grief over the loss of a loved one follows a usual course, as described by psychologists. As the loss recedes into the past, the sharp edges of the pain become a little duller. The memories are more manageable, and life begins to feel more normal.

The grief of infertility does not conform to this pattern, however. Throughout the months and years of diagnostic tests, fertility treatments, and failed efforts to adopt or give birth, the disturbing emotions do not go away; instead they gain in intensity. There may be off times, "vacations" couples take from their efforts. ("I put my Do Not Disturb sign up," one woman told us.) Hope for an answer and optimism about success may ease the grief. But as time goes by, it is harder to sustain this optimism. After five years of trying to conceive, a women wrote to us:

> Infertility is an emotionally devastating disease, which rears its ugly head over and over again. With each month that goes by, the stakes get higher, and the failure is more painful.

Each month without a pregnancy represents less time left to conceive and more evidence of a problem that is not going away. Couples who begin their efforts to have a child in their thirties and are unsuccessful may begin to panic as they see deadlines looming up ahead. Many adoption agencies and IVF programs will not accept women over forty. And there is that internal deadline—the fear of increased risk of birth defects and pregnancy complications.

Resolution may be particularly difficult to obtain for people whose infertility is "unexplained." The frustration can be seen in the following comments:

> It wouldn't be so difficult if I had an answer. I could cope, I could come to terms with myself. Now I can't decide whether I should go another two months for the inseminations, or another six months. What if I don't go? Maybe I would have become pregnant. If I knew, I think I could resign myself to the fact that that's the way things are and look for another option, maybe adoption or childfree living. It hurts deep down inside because I feel like I'm going to live fifty of sixty years and still never know why I never became pregnant. It will always be a mystery.

At each step along the way, couples must ask themselves if it is worth continuing. Some are strengthened in their desire to conceive, more committed than ever. Some parents, even after adopting, are still not ready to stop trying to have a biological child. They are still waiting for a new technique to be developed, still trying an alternative. They love their adopted children, but a resolution of their longing eludes them.

The publicity about new technologies can open the old wounds of those who truly felt they were done with trying to conceive, who had been satisfied for years with their adoptive family. News of IVF babies, tubal transplants, and ovum transfers reawakens old yearnings. Once again they are faced with the uncertainty, with the "what ifs?"

It is difficult to shut the door firmly on biological parenthood. The availability of new technologies makes it a great deal harder. Such technologies are almost impossible to ignore. They offer new hope and what appear to be more choices. But choices such as these can be difficult, shattering the carefully nurtured peace of a family.

Even some of those who feel whole again after a birth or adoption report some residue of sadness. Life is so much better, but it is never the same again.

> I am always aware that my son was conceived with AID and wish he were a joint biological child. But the feeling is not painful and does not hurt my relationship with him or my husband. I feel I have accepted my husband's infertility and our alternatives to it. But I believe I will never forget the situation or stop feeling a little sad.

The struggle does end eventually, one way or another. For many, it ends with a successful birth or births, or it ends with adoption. It may end with a decision that living without children is truly acceptable. The important issue is not how it ends, but how satisfied and comfortable one is with the resolution.

Resolution does not depend on a child or children. While it is very difficult to "give up" the battle and believe it is a positive move, many couples arrive at a point where they can accept there will be no child. They decide they must stop torturing themselves, that their lives can be just as fulfilled in other ways. They are ready to move on. Finally there is peace in their lives.

Whether a couple adopts a child or decides to remain "childfree," it takes great strength to decide to stop trying to conceive. Those who consider stopping have to withstand the urging of their physicians to take the next step. They may have to convince their spouses that they have been through enough. They must repress the "what ifs" in their own minds. When they finally do decide to stop, however, they often experience tremendous relief:

I knew that there was a point when I had to quit. There are just so many times I could allow this kind of invasion, not only into my body, but also into my psyche. I don't know how long you can hang onto the word *hopeful*. You have to come to a time when you say it's over. It was such a relief to put it behind me and get on with my life.

When we asked people if they had any regrets about trying an alternative method of conceiving, 85 percent said no. Yet two major themes emerged again and again in comments about what they wish they had done differently. They regretted, often vehemently, not having sought a fertility specialist earlier. And in many cases they were sorry they had not tried to adopt sooner:

I always believed surgery or IVF would work eventually, and I felt I could only do one thing at a time. Now I wish I would have explored adoption earlier, because time is running out.

People who are able to adopt despite the many obstacles usually discover that the biological connection was not so important after all. As any child grows and develops his or her own independent personality, memories of conception, pregnancy, and birth recede and have little to do with the life of a family. A woman wrote:

It was very important to me to have our own child. But once we adopted a baby, I fell in love with her. All of a sudden I wasn't interested in pursuing in vitro any more.

The birth or adoption of a child brings resolution for many couples. They have achieved their goal of parenthood. Their grief can, at last, be put behind them. If they have a child conceived with the help of an alternative method, the anger they had felt about cost and stress usually disappears. "It was worth every penny," they say. "Anything that important is worth doing whatever you have to do." For other people, adoption brings a happy end to their infertility:

My husband and I have adopted two terrific girls from Korea. I cannot imagine life without the children I have now. They are so much mine that sometimes I can't remember why I was so upset about infertility in the first place.

The Methods

3
Artificial Insemination

Monday morning, ten o'clock. This was by no means a typical day for Cathy and Mark. Each of them had arranged to take the morning off and meet the doctor before his regular office hours. Tense and excited, they hoped that this day would finally mark the successful end of their years of effort and frustration. They felt uncomfortable entering the building, looking over their shoulders and hoping no one would see them. They were surprised to see others in the waiting room—another young couple and several women sitting alone, staring at their magazines. Everyone knew they were all there for the same reason—for artificial insemination.

Mark and Cathy are part of a growing phenomenon, one that has already produced as many as 350,000 babies in the United States.[1] Although artificial insemination has been performed for a long time, until recently it was still rare. There are two kinds of artificial insemination. The semen deposited in a woman, usually with a syringe, may have come from her husband (AIH) or from a donor (AID). Both methods can be used when a man has fertility problems. AIH is also used for some problems that occur in women and for unexplained infertility. AID, because of the involvement of a donor other than the husband, has been much more controversial.

In some ways, donor insemination is a combination of adoption and typical pregnancy, since a couple "adopts" half of the genetic makeup of their child but the woman is still able to have a normal pregnancy and birth. Either kind of artificial insemination allows the man to be present at both the conception and birth and to share the experience of pregnancy just like any other father. It is also the simplest and least expensive form of alternative conception. Because of these advantages and the growing difficulties and higher costs associated with adoption, insemination has become increasingly popular among many infertile couples.

However, one of its advantages—that the child is to all appearances the natural offspring of both parents—may also be the most troublesome aspect. The secrecy surrounding artificial insemination can be a major source of difficulty for the parents. Because of the secrecy, artificial insemination is rarely discussed, and most people are unaware of its availability. When Cathy's physician first suggested it, she was surprised and hesitant; she had never heard of anyone using insemination before.

Mark and Cathy had been married for several years when they decided they were ready to have children. They had been very careful about birth control, wanting to get their careers started before becoming parents. It never occurred to them that they would have any difficulty once they decided to conceive. Yet, after three years of trying, they were beginning to wonder if they would ever have a child. When they both turned thirty, they sought a physicians' advice.

The first thing the doctor did was to test Mark's sperm. It took only a simple test to determine the likely cause of their problem—Mark's sperm count was very low. Both were shocked by the news. They described their feelings:

CATHY: By the time we first went to the doctor, things were already getting bad between us. We were trying so hard to have a baby that our sex life was awful after a while. I didn't want to have anything to do with him—it's not making love, it's just having sex. Then when we learned about his sperm count, well I thought that might finish us altogether. It was really hard for him to accept. But the doctor suggested we try artificial insemination using Mark's sperm, and that gave us both the hope that I could get pregnant. I liked the idea because it would still be our baby.

MARK: When the doctor called with the test results, I just didn't want to believe it. I never thought that not getting pregnant could be my fault. When I first found out about it, I didn't come home for two days. I had to let some steam off so I just went off by myself. I couldn't face Cathy or talk to anyone. It's hard for someone like me to try to explain this to anyone—you know, they'll think you're a deadhead, you can't do anything, you're not really a man. You know every guy looks to have a son. I didn't care so much about my job and making money anymore; I just really wanted to have a family.

I kept asking myself how this could have happened to me. Was it genetic? Maybe I caught VD from someone I had slept with before I met Cathy. Sometimes people say if you masturbate a lot, you'll use it all up. I knew that wasn't true, but I couldn't stop wondering.

AIH and AID: Treatments for Infertility

Traditionally, infertility has been viewed as a woman's problem, with most of the research and tests and treatments directed at the female partner. Yet it is now recognized that abnormalities of the semen are present in 40 to 50 percent of the men in infertile couples. In fact, male sperm count in general has been declining recently, most likely because of environmental causes. Some medical conditions that cause male infertility, such as varicocele (enlargement of a vein in the scrotum), can usually be treated. In many cases, however, there is nothing that can be done to correct the abnormalities that interfere with conception.[2]

The solution for many couples is found in artificial insemination. AIH (insemination with the husband's sperm) may help when the male's sperm count is low or when his sperm have poor motility. In addition, AIH is used for female infertility factors such as poor cervical mucus. It is also possible for either the man or woman to have antibodies that counteract the fertility of otherwise normal sperm; AIH may be used to circumvent this problem. AIH may also be used when a couple has experienced difficulties with intercourse for emotional or physical reasons, or when there has not been a conception for some unknown reason.[3]

The overall success rate of AIH varies greatly from one study to another, depending on the circumstances and method, but the average is about 25 percent. The studies are not well controlled to determine if pregnancy was achieved by AIH or by the couple having normal intercourse. When AIH is performed primarily for a problem with male fertility, there appears to be a much lower than average success rate and possibly a greater likelihood of miscarriage. The Ethics Committee of the American Fertility Society, reflecting on the uncertainty of success in cases of poor sperm count or motility, antibodies, and cervical mucus abnormalities, has recommended that AIH be carried out only in a carefully controlled research setting.[4]

With AIH the husband's sperm is usually deposited in the woman's vagina and lower cervix. An increasing number of doctors put the sperm directly in the uterus. This technique (known as intrauterine insemination) may increase the number of sperm getting to the place of fertilization, but it has disadvantages. It is much more expensive, and there is a small chance of infection. In addition, reports of success rates vary so much that it is difficult to conclude if intrauterine insemination offers a clear advantage over insemination into the vagina.[5]

Donor insemination (AID) is used when the husband has no sperm at all, when there is a severe problem with the number, quality, or motility of the husband's sperm, or when AIH has not worked. If the husband has had a vasectomy, was exposed to toxic materials, or has a history of genetic disease in his family, a couple may turn to AID.[6]

As was true in Mark's case, AIH is often used first, before trying a donor, even though the success rate is fairly low for male factor infertility. For many men, it offers a transition time before the difficult move to the use of a donor. As Mark said:

> I began to think about the doctor's suggestion that we collect my sperm and inseminate Cathy with it. I realized it didn't matter so much to me that the method was unusual, as long as we could still have our baby together. But after five months and still no pregnancy, we were both starting to panic. Having to accept finally that my sperm were useless was the hardest thing I've ever had to do.

Cathy and Mark's physician commented on his approach:

> Husbands using AIH are usually not far along in the process of resolving their feelings. I do AIH many times in preparation for AID because a man might say for instance, "I'll never use another guy's sperm." This way I put the idea in their mind that if you have a lousy sperm count, perhaps you're going to need AID, and even if you don't think it is a reasonable thing, at least you ought to talk about it.

Experts who have studied the impact of insemination on couples recommend that they wait until they have resolved their feelings about the man's infertility before starting AID.[7] For the husband, there is the blow to his sense of himself as a man and a feeling of deficiency in his body. He may feel ashamed that he cannot father a child and regret that he is letting his wife down. Men who think they should be superior and in charge in a relationship may feel deprived and inferior—a source of terrible frustration.

For the wife, there may be anger at her husband, guilt for feeling angry, and guilt that she is fertile when her husband is not. The stress occasionally causes an ordinarily fertile woman to stop ovulating when AID is begun. With both husband and wife feeling angry with themselves and with each other, it is not surprising that conflict and sexual difficulties frequently develop between them. Couples who wait at least a few months after the diagnosis to work through their feelings before starting AID tend to be able to handle the procedure more successfully.

When their doctor suggested donor insemination, Mark and Cathy at first felt they couldn't go through with it. In desperation, they decided to see a counselor to talk through the problems they were facing. Mark said:

> I wanted to have a child so badly, and I also wanted Cathy to be able to experience a pregnancy. But I couldn't stand the idea of my wife carrying somebody else's baby. When the doctor first mentioned it, all I could think was that it would be like another man screwing my wife. I had a hard time explaining my feelings to Cathy, since I was so ambivalent and she seemed eager to try using a donor.
>
> Fortunately, the therapist helped us realize that being a biological father is very different from parenting a child. You leave your mark on the world by the way you parent your child, not by the genes you give him. I still have moments of regret, but I remind myself that AID is just a procedure. Once you have that child, it's yours and you'll love it like it has always been yours.

Not every couple needs a therapist to help them share with each other the feelings they are having. For Mark and Cathy, however, it was helpful. They are now glad they could finally talk together about all of their painful thoughts and emotions before starting insemination. It made it much easier for them to endure the stress of the procedure and to feel that they were working together as a team to reach their goal. Mark is better able to accept his infertility, knowing that Cathy does not love him any less.

The Donor

In addition to having to deal with their grief over Mark's infertility, Mark and Cathy were both concerned about who the donor should be. Just as Mark feared that AID would be like adultery, some people assume that the woman finds a suitable man outside of the marriage and has intercourse with him. One man called a physician known to specialize in artificial insemination in order to volunteer his services—he thought he would be paid for having sex with a woman! When told he could only give a specimen anonymously, he quickly lost interest.

Usually the donor is not known to the couple at all unless they seek him out themselves. In most cases, the physician finds a donor, either through personal contacts or through a sperm bank, and the identity is carefully guarded.

Mark and Cathy were especially concerned about the health of the donor because they knew nothing about him. As Cathy said:

> I was a little leery about the whole thing because you don't really know whose sperm it is. And then I worried a lot about catching AIDS. I know they usually use residents, who I'm sure are in good health, but you just don't know. The doctor said he tries to use people who already had healthy children, and he screens for VD before every insemination.
>
> I think the time I really worried about it the most was when I was pregnant. We both knew a baby is a baby once it's conceived. But you really wonder what the baby is going to be like. You really don't know. We were both shocked when the baby was born healthy.

Who are the donors for artificial insemination? Most donors in the United States are medical students or residents recruited by private physicians for the immediate use of fresh sperm. It has been suggested, in fact, that the term *donor* is misleading since the man is paid for his sperm.

Sperm banks, which tend to recruit a more diverse group of donors, freeze the sperm for future use. A decade ago, as few as 5 percent of all artificial inseminations involved the use of frozen sperm; that figure has probably increased to about 20 percent. Freezing sperm was reported as far back as 1776 in Italy. Ninety years later an Italian pathologist suggested starting a sperm bank so that a woman could produce "legitimate" children in case her husband died on the battlefield. It was not until 1953, however, when new storage techniques were developed, that scientists could thaw sperm without changing its molecular structure. This made it possible to achieve fertilization.[8] With the growing number of sperm banks and further improvements in the freezing procedure, frozen sperm will probably be used even more in the future.

There are advantages and disadvantages involved in using fresh or frozen sperm. Fresh sperm, used the majority of the time, is considerably less expensive and has a higher success rate—about 10 to 15 percent higher than for frozen. The effects of freezing and thawing account for the discrepancy. Yet there are advantages in using frozen sperm. The doctor does not have the problem of finding fresh sperm from a suitable donor within a few hours of the time it is needed. Also, other samples of sperm from the same donor can be used for additional inseminations and can even be used for future pregnancies. Perhaps most important, there is time to test the sperm to detect infectious disease or abnormalities.[9]

The greatest objection voiced by researchers to the present system of sperm donation is the lack of adequate screening. Even though babies born by AID have fewer birth defects than the typical newborn population, there is still great concern about the potential for introducing infections and defective sperm. Most physicians who recruit donors of fresh semen question them only superficially about health and family history, and a donor who is a carrier of a genetic disease may be unaware of this fact. As attorney Lori Andrews, author of *New Conceptions,* writes: "It is ironic that the screening of donor sperm for human AID is much less stringent than that of bull sperm in the cattle industry."[10]

One physician told an especially tragic story of a couple who turned to AID because they were both carriers of Tay-Sachs disease. They had watched their first child die a slow and awful death and did not want to take the chance that another baby would be affected in the same way. What no one knew was that the donor was also a carrier, and the baby born from AID also died from Tay-Sachs.

Another concern about the donors besides their health is the possibility that one man's sperm could be used to inseminate many women, increasing the chance of unwitting marriage between siblings. Although in reality the risks of sibling marriage are still low, it has been estimated that, theoretically, one man could donate enough semen in a year to produce 20,000 children.[11] In fact the pool of donors is usually quite small. One woman commented on this:

> They asked what characteristics we wanted from the donor but warned that special requests might mean a delay since there were so few donors. We often joked that it was probably one guy who went behind a screen and put on a different wig each time depending upon the request.

Because of the potential problems with choosing donors, some couples decide to select their own. A relative of the husband or close friend may be asked, which could allow them to avoid doctors altogether. For the majority of people who prefer not to know the donor, or who cannot find a willing man, experts recommend that people question a physician about the extent of screening and the number of pregnancies that have already resulted from the donor's sperm.

Other experts have also urged the keeping of detailed records of donors. Law professor George Annas argues forcefully that the current practice of discarding all records of the donor's identity ignores the best interests of the child. He calls for sealed records on all AID children and their genetic fathers that would be available to the children when they grow up. Without these records, important information on the medical history of a child is unavailable.[12]

Only about a dozen states now require some form of record keeping, and in one survey, 83 percent of physicians opposed any such legislation.[13] Physicians prefer to control their own practices and not have to respond to legislative requirements. In addition, they seek to protect the confidentiality of donors, many of whom are their colleagues and students.

Many practitioners of AID fear that the requirement of records will scare off potential donors as well as open up a host of possible legal problems. They gain support from the example of Sweden, which passed a law requiring that the donor's identity be recorded and available to children when they turn eighteen.[14] The number of donors dropped dramatically for a while, and couples had to go to other countries for AID. However, the number of donors has increased again, although slowly.

The Experience of Artificial Insemination

In addition to their worry about the donor, Mark and Cathy were apprehensive about the procedure itself. She described what happened:

> Once we decided to try AID, our doctor referred us to a specialist. The first visit was scary. You wonder if people are looking at you because they know what you're there for, especially the nurses. No one ever said anything, of course, but you just wonder what goes on in their heads.
>
> When we met the doctor, he interviewed us both and took a medical history. He asked us if we had any personal preferences and gave us a form to fill out with a lot of personal information, things like the color of our eyes, our hair. He tried to match Mark's height, weight, everything. Then I was told to take my temperature every morning before getting out of bed. When it started to go down, I was to call and get two appointments—one for that day and then one for two days later.
>
> I was really nervous the first time we went for an insemination. Thank God it went more easily than I expected. Mark came with me into the exam room although they didn't really invite him. I was glad he asserted himself because I wanted him there with me. The doctor explained that he was putting a cap over my cervix that had a tube attached to it. It felt a little uncomfortable as he did it. He went in his office for a minute and brought back a container of sperm which had just been delivered by the resident. Then he put a syringe filled with the sperm into the tube that was sticking out of the cap. He folded up the tube so that the sperm would be pushed into the cap. He asked me to stay still for twenty minutes. Then I was instructed how to take out the cap after eight hours.

The procedure for artificial insemination is quite simple, although it varies somewhat from one physician to another. Some, for example, do not use a cervical cap as Cathy's doctor did, especially when using frozen sperm. Some use a drug to stimulate ovulation, but many do not. Physicians may inseminate two or three times a month. Some couples pick up frozen sperm from their physician and perform the insemination at home by themselves.

Many couples who have been through AIH or AID now wish they had done it at home, if possible. In that way they could have avoided some of the difficulties that arise when coordinating with the physician's schedule. More important, it would have been less impersonal, and the husband could have been actively involved. The procedure is fairly simple. By using a syringe bought in a drug store, semen is transferred from a container to the vagina. Some physicians will teach couples how to do this if they ask for instruction.

Many times couples request that the husband's sperm be mixed with the donor's or decide to have intercourse just before or after the insemination. They hope in this way to maintain the possibility that any child conceived could be the husband's. Many physicians, however, recommend against the mixing of sperm and urge couples to refrain from intercourse prior to insemination. Sperm from different men can sometimes negate each other's effectiveness, and the success rate seems to be higher when there is no mixing.[15]

Cathy went home after the first insemination feeling very excited. She felt sure she must be pregnant. She said:

> It felt like magic—the electricity in my belly. I was so sure I was pregnant that it was like losing a baby when I found out I wasn't. Because it didn't work the first time, I would protect myself and say "No, I'm not pregnant" and just feel it's not going to happen. I thought that this is something I'm going to do every month for the rest of my life and I'm never going to get pregnant. One month I broke the thermometer, partly on purpose. I was starting to get very depressed about this.

It is not unusual for a couple to experience frustration and depression when insemination fails to produce a pregnancy quickly. Particularly after so many years of difficulty in achieving a pregnancy, AID may be seen as a last resort. If it does not succeed, despair can set in, and many couples abandon the effort after a few months. Yet persistence may pay off, and most physicians recommend that, if a couple can afford it, at least six months of insemination be tried before considering other options.[16]

Studies of AID report an average success rate of 60 percent, although in different studies they range from 37 to 84 percent. Martin Curie-Cohen and colleagues, in the most complete national study yet done, found that those physicians who did the most inseminations also had the highest success rate.[17]

After seven months of inseminations, Cathy and Mark were discouraged and upset. The costs of the procedure were mounting. Although artificial insemination usually costs far less than IVF (in vitro fertilization) or hiring a surrogate, the monthly expenses mount up quickly. Each time a woman is inseminated, there is the charge for the office visit and the fee for the sperm sample. In addition, she may be taking expensive fertility drugs to stimulate her ovulation. If a couple uses intrauterine insemination, the visit is more expensive, and there is often a charge for washing and preparing the sperm. The people we interviewed said they were spending anywhere from $100 to $600 a month for artificial insemination.

The emotional strain was even more difficult for Mark and Cathy than the financial burden. Cathy said:

> It was very hard on us. The fear that it might not work was always there. I felt the emptiness would be endless and all this effort would be futile. All the waiting each month was so hard. Another problem for both of us was the hassle of leaving work and making up enough excuses so that there would not be too many questions and then pray that I had chosen the right day.

The next month Cathy became pregnant. Mark was very excited and involved in the pregnancy. They both worried though about what the baby was going to look like. Cathy tried not to think about the donor, but sometimes she dreamed it was the doctor. Other times she had moments of panic that the donor was really totally different from Mark, and maybe even from another nationality or race. Most of the time, though, she felt overwhelmed with gratitude to this unknown person who had made it possible for her to become a mother.

People who have used AID report widely differing feelings toward the donor. Some wish they could meet him and see what he looks like or thank him for his help. Others dismiss the donor, saying they have purchased a product and the person behind it is irrelevant to them. Most people know they will never be able to find out who the donor is and prefer to try to forget about him.

When Cathy and Mark's baby, Michael, was born, they were both ecstatic to be parents at last. All of the worries they had had seemed insignificant. When asked if they have any sense of how the method of conception might affect their relationship to Michael, who is now five years old, they replied:

CATHY: When Michael was very young, I stepped back and let Mark do things more than I would have otherwise, because I feel I have this genetic claim on him and Mark is going to need to have something special to make up for that. Over the years this has changed and I feel we are more equal about everything.

MARK: I am his father—there is no doubt in my mind. As he's growing and his features are getting more definite, I wonder who else has a nose like that. But these feelings are minor compared to the joy and gratitude of having him.

Keeping AID Secret

For most parents, the joy of having and raising a healthy child far outweighs any problems that might accompany AID. However, there are some problems faced by parents. One of these is the feeling they have done something deviant, something not really accepted by others. According to Bernard Rubin, who reviewed the history of artificial insemination, it has been discussed as far back as the second century and practiced since at least 1793. He reports, however, that it has always been opposed from many sides.[18]

In the past, some physicians called the procedure "socially monstrous," "an offense against society." Courts ruled that AID is a form of adultery and the children born from it "illegitimate." Leaders of many religious groups have forbidden its use, claiming that it would endanger the family and violate religious precepts. Pope Pius XII, in voicing the Catholic church's opposition in 1949, claimed that AID would "convert the domestic hearth, sanctuary of the family, into nothing more than a biological laboratory."[19]

This opposition has mostly disappeared. The medical profession now openly accepts and endorses AID, and the courts and legislatures in many states have passed laws to ensure that the children have the same status as any other child born to a married couple. Sperm banks have multiplied, and infertility is a subject openly discussed in the media and among many couples. AID is increasingly available to single heterosexual and lesbian women as well as to married couples. Apparently many of the legal, medical, and psychological obstacles have been overcome in the last two decades.

But that does not mean going through with the procedure is easy, that there are not a host of emotional as well as medical and legal problems remaining. The Catholic church as well as the most conservative of Jewish and Protestant leaders are still opposed.[20] The general public is largely uninformed and unsupportive.

Secrecy is a key issue for those involved in insemination. Artificial insemination is almost always surrounded by secrecy— secrecy about the identity of the donor, secrecy between the couple and their friends and family about what they are doing, and secrecy from the child conceived about his or her true origins. The first recorded case of successful AID, in 1884, was done during an examination of the woman without telling the couple involved. Since then, according to sociologist Robert Snowden and colleagues, some physicians have advocated, if possible, not telling the husband that he is infertile or that a donor is going to be used.[21]

Most physicians and other staff members of AID programs strongly encourage their patients to keep AID a secret from everyone. They even suggest not telling the obstetrician who delivers the baby, so that the husband's name will be put on the birth certificate as father without hesitation. As one woman said:

> The doctor told us it's nobody else's business, that it's just between the two of us and him, and no one else has to know. That was a hard thing, you know, because so many times you want to say it. It's a hard thing to explain, and people seem to think that if you can't have your own, you shouldn't have any or you should adopt. I have a feeling his

parents wouldn't accept the baby if they knew. They wouldn't think she was a part of him.

The secrecy inevitably produces some awkwardness at times, especially when family members and friends speculate, as they always do, about which parent a child resembles. One father recalled:

When he was little, everyone said he looked just like me. My mother has a picture of me when I was little and she held it up against him and she said they looked identical, like twins. I used to say, "No, look how different he looks," but now I just play along with it—I know what really happened.

Most couples feel torn between a desire to keep the information private and a strong need to talk to others about it. They are fearful of others' reactions. Yet they also talk about the stress of "living a lie" and the wish to share such an important event with those to whom they are close. Some wish they could meet others who have also used AID so they could compare their feelings and experiences.

No matter how strongly they expressed a commitment to secrecy, most of the people in our study had told at least one or two others. They were selective, often telling one set of parents but not the other, or certain friends they assumed would be sympathetic. But they have found it difficult not to tell anyone at all.

The central dilemma for parents is whether or not to tell their children. The great majority of parents who used AID insist that they will never reveal the circumstances of the conception to their children.[22] By not informing the child, the parents need never worry about a later search for the identity of the biological father. More important, they feel they will avoid any stigma that they or the child might suffer for seeming "abnormal." After all, they reason, why create unnecessary problems, particularly if friends and relatives also do not know and therefore the risk of a child's hearing from other sources is minimal?

Certainly most parents who conceive "naturally" do not tell children about the circumstances of their conception. Unlike the adopted child, where others know and neither of the parents is involved genetically, the child born of AID appears to be the product of the parents' normal pregnancy and birth. As one father said:

I couldn't tell him. You know, I will have raised him all his life and I just wouldn't have the heart to tell him. I'm afraid he'd be ashamed of me. It might break my heart as well as his.

Then why tell the children? Some experts claim it is essential that children know their medical history and not assume they may share any medical problems experienced by the fathers who raised them. Some also fear that maintaining a secret about the child's origin is ultimately unhealthy for the family. Aphrodite Clamar, writing in the *American Journal of Psychoanalysis*, emphasizes this possibility: "By its very nature, a secret is a potent force, assuming undue proportion and power within the family—an existential fact that remains unspoken, yet controls and colors the lives of the people involved."[23] Children may sense that something is being hidden from them. Those who are eventually told often feel relieved because they had guessed that there was something different, or bad, about themselves.

The physicians who provide AID usually counsel silence; social scientists who have studied AID almost always encourage openness. With the experts disagreeing and compelling arguments on both sides, parents are faced once more with a dilemma created by the benefits of technology. (See Chap. 10 for further discussion.)

Single Heterosexual and Lesbian Women

Single heterosexual and lesbian women who want very much to have children are turning more and more to AID as a solution.[24] Either they do not want intimacy with a man or prefer to avoid problems by not knowing the identity of the father. As one lesbian woman said:

Sex with somebody that I'm not involved with otherwise would seem so mercenary. It wasn't anything I ever considered. I kind of liked the idea of having a virgin birth. And anyway, conception is conception, it's just a matter of how the sperm gets there.

Many single heterosexual women who seek out AID hope to get married but cannot wait any longer to find the right man before having children. As difficult as it is for married couples to adopt, it is even more so for unmarried women. AID is then an attractive alternative. A single mother of a four-year-old son born by AID talked about her situation:

> It's hard raising a child by yourself. But my family has been wonderful. My parents were concerned at first about the man and what he does and what he looks like. But they loved the baby from the moment he was born—it just doesn't matter anymore where the sperm came from. It's also helpful that I have friends who did the same thing, and our kids will be friends with each other and not feel so unusual.

The most difficult problem faced by unmarried women is obtaining AID. Many physicians and clinics refuse to inseminate anyone who is not in a stable marriage, and public attitudes are still unsympathetic. It is necessary, therefore, for single women to seek out a physician or a sperm bank willing to help them, or simply to do the insemination themselves.

A lesbian couple who had used a turkey baster to inseminate one partner received a great deal of media attention when they split up and the other partner sued for visitation rights. While the story created a sensation in the press, it is not an isolated case. In fact, information regarding techniques of home insemination has moved quickly through networks of lesbian women seeking to avoid the difficulties (and expense) of approaching physicians.

Despite the growing number of children conceived by the artificial insemination of unmarried women, it has been estimated that they still comprise only about 1 percent of all inseminations.[25] This proportion is certain to increase, but the obstacles point to the control that many physicians have over access to this technology. It is an example of the medical profession's enforcement of social mores in the dispensing of services.

♦   ♦   ♦   ♦   ♦

Studies of families that have undergone artificial insemination have uncovered very few significant problems as a result, and one study even found that AID couples have a much lower divorce rate than average.[26] Perhaps the process of working through the conflicts of infertility leads to stronger relationships in those who have had AID. Most families are very positive about the results, and many return to be inseminated for a second child. These results have contributed to a more open-minded attitude on the part of those physicians and lawmakers who recognize the benefits for infertile families.

Not everyone is as fortunate as Mark and Cathy, who did finally have a child with AID. Those people for whom AIH or AID does not work are confronted with new decisions. What should they do next? Depending on the nature of the problem, they may try another method. Many couples, for example, who used AIH for female or unexplained infertility and for whom, therefore, AID is not appropriate, consider whether to try IVF or other treatments. Many others look into adopting a child.

For those who do succeed, artificial insemination, like many of the new technologies, creates dilemmas for individual families to resolve. It is certain to become increasingly common and more successful and therefore probably more public. Even so, it is likely to remain a secretive process, one producing a very private, but troubling, joy for parents. As Cathy said:

> I don't really think about it anymore. Just once in a while I wonder what other people would think if they knew and what Michael would think if he knew. I wonder how other parents who have had AID deal with it. And then I forget about it again, and we're just like any other family.

4
In Vitro
Fertilization

*We flew into the Norfolk, Virginia, airport, coming in
low over the ocean with its persistent, lapping waves.
It was a beautiful warm day, a day we had looked
foward to for two years. I was one determined lady to
get pregnant, even if it meant a long wait to get into
what we considered the best in vitro program in the
country. I was going to force a baby out of my body; it
meant so much to me. As we rode in a cab to the
Medical Tower, I wondered how many thousands of
others had already made this same trip, this "pilgrimage
to Mecca." Were they all as filled with nervous
excitement as I was, as desperate and as hopeful? How
many had left again by the same route, their dreams
destroyed in sunny Norfolk? I prayed that I would be
one of the lucky ones.*
                                        —Jane, an IVF mother

Tens of thousands of people, like this woman, are now considering *in vitro fertilization* (IVF). The birth of Louise Brown, the
first "test-tube baby" in England in 1978, represented a major
breakthrough in fertility treatment, drawing the attention of the
world to the miracle of IVF. The first American program opened
in Norfolk, Virginia, in 1981, and well over a hundred more have
followed. Worldwide, at least three thousand babies have already
been born as a result of this method.[1]

The growing availability of IVF has raised many questions. Is it the most promising new technology, helping those who cannot conceive to fulfill their dreams? Or does it offer false hope to people who are willing to try anything to have a baby?

There is no doubt that it is controversial. The image of scientists creating human embryos in a laboratory is frightening to many people. They see IVF as leading to dangerous manipulations of life. But for those couples who seek out IVF, the controversies are irrelevant. They have spent years trying to have a biological child, and they often believe IVF is their last hope. Even though it may reopen a Pandora's box of anxieties and grief once thought resolved and despite the fact that it is difficult, expensive, stressful, and unlikely to succeed, each couple sustains the hope that for them, at least, it will produce a miracle.

Carol and Tim have been searching for this miracle for almost ten years. For years their lives have been dominated by temperature charts and sex on schedule. Carol has been through multiple tests with several doctors. She has had surgery twice and has taken fertility drugs. For Carol and Tim, IVF is not a radical new experiment. It is simply the last of a long series of intrusive and difficult procedures. It is the end of the line for them.

During these years, Tim has worked hard to built up his own business and Carol has been enjoying a successful career. Yet their minds were never far from their preoccupation with becoming parents. Carol said:

> I had all the usual tests done—everything from A to Z. After years of tests and two operations, the end result was absolutely nothing—unexplained infertility. I went to another infertility specialist to get a second opinion and was told, "Relax, keep trying." They couldn't find anything. I always thought they were implying that the problem was in my mind, and, although I didn't think so, I would wonder. It's the 1980s; they should be able to come up with something tangible. It's like I'm out on a limb, I'm in limbo somewhere.
>
> I kept thinking I had to do something, find more information, see other doctors, or else nothing would happen. It was so frustrating to keep calling and writing people, because it takes so much emotional energy to do

that. But I did it anyway because I wanted a baby so badly. Finally, one doctor suggested I try in vitro. He referred me to a medical center about an hour from our home that had recently started a program.

For some lucky couples, fewer than 10 percent of those who start the process, IVF succeeds with the birth of a baby. For all those who fail to become pregnant, or who have miscarriages or ectopic pregnancies, it brings renewed stress and grief. For many, it is the final procedure that closes their struggle for a biological child.

The great majority of people in our study who had tried IVF felt it was worth the effort. They might have been angry at a specific program, and they might have been unhappy if the procedure did not work. But despite all of the stress, almost no one was sorry at least to have tried.

When IVF was first developed, it was intended primarily as a way of bypassing damaged or blocked fallopian tubes. As infertility specialists became more experienced with the techniques of IVF, many clinics began to extend it to couples with other problems such as endometriosis (when pieces of the uterine lining attach to the tubes or ovaries and prevent conception), male infertility, poor sperm-mucus interaction, and unexplained infertility such as Carol and Tim experienced.[2]

The major purpose of IVF has been to join the egg of a woman to the sperm of her husband so that they could produce a biological child together. Eggs are removed from a woman's ovary, usually by a surgical procedure called a laproscopy, and fertilized with the husband's sperm in a small shallow container called a petri dish. After waiting two days to see if the cells have divided, the physician inserts the fertilized eggs through the woman's vagina into her uterus.[3]

As IVF has been perfected and gained greater public acceptance, physicians have begun to offer a number of variations to couples with more complex problems. A woman with damaged tubes whose husband has a low or absent sperm count can now have her eggs fertilized in the petri dish by a donor's sperm. If a woman's ovaries are missing or inaccessible, she may receive donated eggs which are fertilized by her husband. Or if she can produce an egg but for some reason cannot carry a baby, the couple's embryo may be transferred to a surrogate mother.[4]

Success Rates

One of the first questions most couples ask as they are investigating IVF is the likelihood of success. They usually are told that the success rate is between 20 percent and 30 percent. This number can be misleading. It does not take into account the chances of success for the couple's specific conditions or age-group. For example, couples with male infertility problems or unexplained infertility do not appear to do as well as those whose difficulty comes from blocked fallopian tubes or endometriosis. The statistics also often reflect a national rate gathered from the most experienced clinics, ignoring the fact that the particular clinic where a couple is seeking help may have had no success at all. In fact, a recent survey by the American Fertility Society found that one-third of all IVF clinics in the United States had never had a successful birth.[5]

It is very difficult to state an actual rate of success. Some IVF programs define success as a positive pregnancy test while others wait for a visible fetus on ultrasound exam at six weeks. Yet as many as half of IVF pregnancies will result in ectopic pregnancies or miscarriages. Close monitoring of the woman may produce an early diagnosis of what is called a "chemical pregnancy," one that aborts so early that in unmonitored women it would not be recognized. It is also hard to give an exact rate because at any given time there are people who are in the middle of the process, waiting to start another attempt, or currently pregnant. Many drop out after one or two tries. Therefore, clinics usually present their rates as the number of pregnancies compared to the total number of laparoscopies or to the number of embryo transfers.[6]

The most crucial question, the best measure of success, is how many couples that entered a program actually ended up with babies. The answer to that question is considerably lower than 20 percent. Our survey of American IVF programs in 1985–86 showed that the percentage of couples who started IVF and actually had a successful birth ranged from 0 percent to 30 percent, with most programs having birth rates below 10 percent.

The extent to which some clinics mislead people in reporting their success rates can be seen in a letter to us from one center reporting one birth and three current pregnancies out of almost one hundred patients. At best this would be a 4 percent success rate. Yet this clinic, continuing its report, claimed a 20 percent pregnancy rate with 50 percent ending in miscarriages. Another program that had had no pregnancies after several attempts was featured in a local newspaper report with the claim that success could be achieved as often as 50 percent of the time. As more and more new programs open around the country, there is greater competition for patients, which certainly increases the incentive for a clinic to claim a good success rate.

Those who can afford IVF do not appear to be discouraged by the low success rates. They hope to defy the odds, to prove that this high-stakes gamble will pay off for them. They may be deceiving themselves. In order to begin a program such as IVF, it may be necessary to ignore accurate information about the very low rates of success. Even when the poor chances of having a baby from IVF are carefully presented in advance, couples often do not believe what they hear. A nurse coordinator in an IVF program described this mental screening process:

> The majority of patients are very well read. They know that one place may have a 20 percent success rate, and we have a rate of 10 percent. But for them it's never 10 percent or 20 percent, they all believe that their own chance of having a baby is 50 percent or 70 percent or 80 percent. Maybe they have to believe that to come here.

Physicians and patients alike engage in magical thinking about the possibility of having a baby. Staff members of new programs are convinced that they will achieve high success rates, and they communicate this to couples. A woman who had already been through IVF three times describes how she convinced herself that her chances were good despite the evidence:

> The doctor told me that I was the twelfth woman in the program. He didn't want to tell me if they had had any successes yet, but I kept asking. I wanted to know what my odds were. He had already told me that the chance of implantation was one in seven. When he finally said that they had had no successes yet, I felt really good, it increased my high. I figured if there had already been one in the first group of seven, then the next one would be number fourteen instead of number twelve. This way it felt like my chances were better.

Many people decide not to take the risk of trying IVF; for them the low success rates are too discouraging. For example, of the women who wrote in our questionnaire that they had considered IVF, more than one-third said they had rejected the idea because of the poor success rates.

Advocates of IVF point out that the natural conception rate is also low. Even fertile people who have intercourse during ovulation have only a one-in-four chance of conceiving. Some physicians claim that IVF can match and may ultimately exceed the natural pregnancy rate. This remains to be seen.[7]

A recent technique, referred to as GIFT (gamete intrafallopian transfer), may achieve greater success than the usual IVF procedure because it makes it possible in some cases for fertilization to occur within the woman's body instead of in the laboratory. As soon as the eggs are retrieved by laporoscopy, they are immediately mixed with the man's semen and returned to the fallopian tube. Physicians hope for a higher success rate when fertilization takes place in its normal site, but this is possible only for a woman who has at least one healthy tube.[8]

Carol described her experience of learning about the possibility of success with IVF:

> During our first interview, we spoke to a doctor and the nurse coordinator. They were extremely nice and supportive and gave us detailed information about the procedure and what to expect. They told us that the success rate for this procedure was about 17 percent. At that time I didn't realize that they hadn't had any successes at all, and that they had been doing it for only six months.
>
> I would have done it even if I had known that. At least it was a chance and if I didn't do it I would never know whether I had that chance or not. Also I liked the fact that it was one of the newer programs because I thought that we would get more attention. It made it seem like we were doing something important, something that probably not too many people in this area go through.

The Experience of IVF

The IVF procedure is based on precise timing and continuous monitoring of the woman's responses. For several weeks the woman's life is dominated by injections of fertility drugs, ultrasounds, blood tests, followed by surgery and more blood tests. Carol described the procedure and the physical and emotional difficulties it entailed:

After our initial interview, we waited three months before the start of the procedure. It was really very hard once we started. I think because you want this so badly and try to protect yourself from the hope, especially after so many disappointments, you begin to feel you can't do it. But somehow we kept going.

Tim started giving me the Pergonal injections on the third day of my cycle in order to help produce more than one egg. The shots were a little scary, but the main thing is that I felt I couldn't escape what we were doing. I couldn't try to distract myself or pretend this wasn't happening. I was dragged right into it because I was so physically involved for the entire month.

On the sixth day I started going to the hospital for ultrasounds. Each morning I would sit in the waiting room with other couples, drinking water to fill up my bladder, so that they could see if follicles [the sacs in which eggs develop] were growing on my ovaries. They would say you have three follicles, sized 1.2, 1.4, and 1.7. I kept thinking, am I going to make it? My blood, my numbers, are they going to find follicles? Will they be big enough? Will I make it to the laparoscopy?

At every stage I was terrified that I would fail and not make it to the next step. I was scared and upset, but I was afraid to show my feelings or go to the counselor there. I thought they might ask me to leave the program because I wasn't handling it well. There was also the feeling that I didn't want to say anything because I would be jinxed.

Then they told me the time looked good to release the eggs from the follicles. To do this they stopped the fertility drugs and gave me an injection of HCG [Human Chorionic Gonadotropin, a substance that completes egg maturation and can trigger the release of the eggs from the follicles thirty to forty hours after it is injected]. It really drew me in when I saw those eggs on the surface of my ovary in the ultrasound.

A day and a half later, I went into surgery for the removal of the eggs. When I woke up, the doctor told me they had gotten three eggs and they looked pretty good. I felt a tremendous sense of relief at that point. The worst part physically was over—the ultrasounds, the driving back and forth, and then the surgery.

The anesthesia made me sick for a while. While I was vomiting in the recovery room, Tim wanted to know where I thought he should go and masturbate to give his sperm. I couldn't believe it. I just told him to take his *Penthouse* magazine and go find a bathroom. They told me that they took Tim's semen to the lab, washed it, separated the sperm from the fluid, and placed it in an incubator for several hours. Then a lab technician placed a few drops of the most active sperm onto each egg to fertilize it.

Not everyone who starts IVF gets as far as Carol did, since there are several points in the procedure at which something may not work. For some women (5–20 percent), when a screening laparoscopy is performed, it reveals inaccessible ovaries, and the couple either is eliminated from the program, attempts ultrasound-guided egg retrieval, or must consider using a donor's eggs if they are available. Of the women who do continue and who go through the drug therapy, 10 to 30 percent discover that the egg follicles have not developed sufficiently or cannot be retrieved. When eggs are removed, about 10 percent of the time they fail to fertilize.[9] As one woman who never got to the laparoscopy said:

I'd been there for a week and things were not looking very good. The eggs were not developing the way they wanted them to. That was hard to take. Here the nurse is telling everybody after the ultrasounds to come back tomorrow. Then she sits down quietly in the corner with me and says, "Well, we're sorry to have to scrap this cycle." It was like someone had died.

Carol felt fortunate to be among those who made it through all of the initial stages. She said:

I burst into tears when the nurse called and told me eggs had divided. I realized I had finally created new life.

Two days after surgery, I went back for the embryos to be transferred into my uterus. When they put them in with the fluid, I was scared to move. I had to stay on my hands and knees with my rear end elevated for the transfer—all of this with eight people looking at me. What a humiliating position. But I guess I'm beyond embarrassment at this point.

It was also *very* exciting. It tasted like hope—real hope. My body was all puffed up from the Pergonal shots and I felt pregnant. I knew a live embryo was in my uterus. This was the closest I had ever been to being pregnant. Then the two-week wait to see if an embryo would implant, and I would be officially pregnant. After one week my hopes were the highest, but I could barely endure the strain of waiting, thinking every twinge from my waist down was either menstrual cramps or early signs of pregnancy.

Then during the second week, I felt I was getting my period. That awful roller coaster we had been living on was coming crashing down again.

The nurse called with the results of the first blood test I took to check for pregnancy. She said it looked good but inconclusive. When I went for the next blood test, the staff were all excited. Maybe I'd be their first success. My hopes were soaring again.

Then they called and told me the latest blood test was negative. Even though I half expected it, I was devastated. I didn't realize how much it would affect me. I thought I was handling it real well, but I couldn't even talk to them.

All those feelings I thought had been resolved came right back again. We had never been so close to a pregnancy—never quite felt this hopeful before. That made it painful. For weeks I lay awake at night trying to visualize those embryos inside of me, trying to figure out why it didn't work.

Tim shared in the terrible disappointment:

The day we heard the news I couldn't believe it. I didn't want to believe it. All my rational sense of the poor probabilities didn't prevent us from feeling that we had just lost a baby. I started to focus on work intensely. I couldn't stand to see Carol's pain—I didn't want to see her cry.

The news of failure after weeks of intense effort and hope is crushing. It is compounded for many by a sense of abandonment, a break in the close and constant contact that binds couples to clinic staff and to others going through the program. One IVF counselor described this rupture:

You call a patient and tell her that you have a negative pregnancy test, the phone call is over, but you know somebody at the end of the line is falling apart. There needs to be some real hand-holding at that time because of the emotional feeling that somehow the patient has failed, and the medical team feels that way too. That's one of the reasons we have a hard time dealing with it, because we too have failed.

The intense daily relationship between staff and patient is over, often ending without even a good-bye. This breaking off of communication, a frequent occurrence, is particularly hard on couples because they are grieving. They grieve for those living growing embryos that should have become babies and instead died in the woman's body.

"Some women become attached to those embryos in a way that's very similar to how attached women get to a pregnancy," explained a psychologist who counsels infertile couples. "They are really experiencing a failed cycle of in vitro as a miscarriage." Just as with a miscarriage, couples may go through intense feelings of depression and anger. They may feel guilty; once again they may blame themselves for having done something wrong or simply for being inadequate. They may be jealous of others who have achieved pregnancies by IVF or who have never had to struggle with infertility.

Despite the trauma they had just experienced, Carol and Tim reminded each other that they had originally agreed to try the procedure at least three times. They figured they would devote one year to in vitro. At that point Carol would be thirty-five, and they would then decide what to do next. Carol explained:

In my head I knew it made sense to try it again. I thought, I've endured one loss and I know what that's like. It's very painful, but it didn't kill me. My choice is to try one or two more times with the months of grief attached to it, and maybe have a success, or not to try at all. As hard as it was, knowing that we got so far gave me hope to try again. Maybe the next time would be lucky for us. I'm glad I did it. I don't think I could have rested, knowing that the technology existed, until I had tried it. It was painful, but so were the other years of my life that I was trying to get pregnant. Those were my choices. I could quit or I could try.

Tim was also ready to try again:

Two months later we were back. It was easier the second time because we knew everybody there and knew what was involved. The part that made the first one hard was not knowing your way around the medical center and feeling bounced from one lab or office to another. You also don't know whether you're going to drop out at any point. They come up with all sorts of little traps along the way and give you only little pieces of information as you go along. I would think we've made it and then find out that no, that was just one piece and there's still another step to be done. We got through all the steps the first time; so I was very positive about our chances of being successful if we tried again.

I was so excited when they told me that this time they retrieved eleven eggs from Carol. They were very encouraging. I felt like we got 100 on a test and this was the time it was going to happen for us.

The development of follicles, eggs, and embryos become very important psychological steps for couples going through IVF. As Carol observed:

You go for these tests and you bring the results back to the nurse there, the picture of the follicles, which wasn't always very encouraging. She'd say, "Is that all there is? Come on Carol, you gotta get them bigger." What did she think? Of course, I would like to make them as big as possible!

Carol and Tim felt sure that since there were so many eggs retrieved this time, they were going to make it. When the results of the final blood test were negative, they were devastated again. Carol said:

I was afraid I was going crazy, especially after I got my period. I couldn't go to work and I couldn't stop crying. Again I felt like I had lost a baby, but it would sound strange to tell that to my friends and family. So I couldn't share the feelings very well. There were several months of mourning when nothing else in life seemed worthwhile. I felt physically depleted, not to mention seeing all this money thrown out the window for nothing. We had very little left. I really wanted to run away from it all.

But at the same time, I realized that it hadn't been all negative. At least, after all these years of trying to get pregnant, we knew we could make an embryo. That was one step further along. And the doctors were still encouraging—they hadn't given up.

A positive aspect of the IVF experience for Carol and Tim was Tim's involvement in the procedure. Tim commented:

I felt more actively involved with the in vitro than with any other part of the infertility procedures. Maybe because I became so involved, I was very hopeful. I thought I was going to faint when I had to give Carol the first shot. I always had a phobia about needles. But it really made me appreciate what Carol was going through physically. Then watching the ultrasounds, watching Carol go into surgery one more time, was really hard. I admired Carol's courage. I don't think I could go through the same thing.

Many couples feel that IVF gives them an opportunity for greater control over the procedure, while others are glad to be told what to do and not worry about control. The programs vary a great deal in how much they involve couples, such as the man giving Pergonal shots to the woman, or the couple taking samples to the lab. But ultimately the outcome is out of their hands. As one infertility counselor noted:

They make the decision to do it. But are they going to be accepted in the program? That's out of their control. It's all of these hurdles they have to leap over. There's the whole process of inducing ovulation. Then the laparoscopy being done under general anesthesia is the ultimate in loss of control and powerlessness. I think the only control they really have is deciding which program, how many times they will try, how they're going to cope as a couple, and how they're going to utilize their network of family and friends.

Carol and Tim had agreed to try three times, and although they were feeling very discouraged, they decided to stick to their original plan. By this time they knew the ropes and they were feeling close to some of the staff. Tim recalled:

As much as it had been difficult, and they weren't always equipped to meet our needs, we still felt that they were like family. You can get to know people pretty well in those circumstances. One of the doctors was really super, and we also came to rely on the nurse coordinator a lot. When things got really tough for us after the second cycle, we went to see the social worker at the clinic, and she was a big help.

For some couples, trouble arises because one member of the couple is more interested in pursuing IVF than the other. Often the husband feels that he is just going along to keep his wife happy, but that it is really her project. Some men are reluctant to see their wives subjected to yet another series of tests and treatment. When the two are not in agreement, a failed IVF attempt may produce a great deal of anger and mutual blaming.

. Some IVF programs have a full-time social worker who offers counseling and organizes support groups. Others use a therapist only at the beginning in order to help couples talk about their feelings about infertility and any ambivalence they have about IVF. However, since these interviews are part of the initial screening, many people are reluctant to speak openly for fear of being dropped from the program. In reality, it is very rare for the therapist to recommend that a couple be excluded, and the assessment is intended rather to help couples and alert the staff to any special problems of which they should be aware.[10]

Most programs offer no counseling at all. As one director said:

> We take pride—we do a good job of talking to people. I don't think we do as good a job for someone who really has a more pronounced need, but it's like a lot of other things with an IVF program—someone's got to pay for it, and I think the expense is prohibitive.

For many couples, the contacts they have with clinic staff are all they need, but many more with whom we talked expressed a desire for more counseling as part of the program. Some felt they were treated very impersonally; although they were not sorry to have tried IVF, they were angry at the staff. As one man said:

> You know, we've been infertile a long time and we finally get to this fancy medical center and pretty soon we realized that these guys were only spending ten minutes with us if we were lucky. We just weren't getting our questions answered, and of course it wasn't working either. It was just so frustrating. The whole process is so much black magic. You get the impression you're part of an experiment, a little cog in their big machine, just another one of fifty people being herded like sheep through exactly the same thing with no personal interest in you as an individual.

Part of this anger is an inevitable component of the grief from failure. The clinics that make efforts to offer personalized care and support may be better able than the others to help couples through this difficult process. They are certainly more appreciated. But this kind of support is highly unusual.

One important source of support is the other couples who are going through IVF at the same time. Tim described the bond he felt to these other couples:

> They were mostly people like us, in their thirties, educated, and from middle- or upper-middle-class areas. They had all been through infertility problems for many years. All these women had their battle scars from surgeries, and their bodies had been probed and prodded. All the guys had jerked off a million times in the bathroom. With all of these things we had in common, there was a lot of mutual support.

There may be a certain amount of competition among people in the same cycle (e.g., who has the biggest eggs?), but ordinarily this is greatly outweighed by the help. These couples sometimes stay in touch with each other long after their connection with the center has ended.

Even before Carol and Tim received that last phone call informing them once again of a negative pregnancy test after their third attempt, they had the feeling that it was all over for them with IVF. They knew they would have to accept that they were unlikely to have a biological child. Carol was glad that at least it was over:

> When the third time failed, I felt exhausted, I was angry and upset, but part of me felt like it was over and that was a relief. I knew I had done it all and now I could stop, I was tired. By the time we finished in vitro, I had come to the point where the need to have a biological child had been beaten out of me. I had wanted desperately to be pregnant with our own child. Inch by inch I started to give up that need, and I felt I was ready to consider adoption.

For many couples who do not succeed, IVF can lead to closure. They feel that they have tried everything and now can begin to accept the fact that they are not going to be able to have a child together. Carol and Tim went through the procedure three times before they could come to this point. Couples sometimes reach this resolution after one time, while others are unwilling to give up even after six or more trials.

Many couples have to drop out of the program because it is simply too expensive to go on. The cost of each cycle is usually $4,000 to $5,000, and many insurance companies do not cover

IVF. There are the additional expenses of transportation, lodging, and food if one uses a center away from home. Because of these high costs, many people cannot even try one time, and others make great sacrifices for this chance. Some people feel it really isn't a choice—"We do what we have to do," they say. Another woman agreed:

> You pay your money and take your chances. What good is money if you don't have the thing you want most—to have children?

Other people express a great deal of anger and resentment about having to spend so much, especially when the procedure fails. One man voiced his opinion:

> The price tag is outrageous! These programs are entirely too expensive. Why should people have to go to the poorhouse simply to exercise their inalienable right of having a child?

For many people the "price tag" makes the decision for them. They may buy lottery tickets in the hope of some day winning a large sum, but in the meantime they simply cannot afford to go on. In our survey, we found that people with little insurance coverage who made less than about $40,000 per year could not afford to try IVF at all. Money is also the major reason given by the many who stop IVF after one cycle.

In a survey of 121 patients who withdrew from an in vitro program after one attempt, two main reasons were given for leaving. Financial burdens was one. The other major problem was the stress of the procedure. People mentioned the tremendous anxiety, depression, disruption of work or career, and strain on their marriages.[11]

Despite the cost and stress, many couples find it hard to stop. They are encouraged by the programs to keep going. Sitting in the waiting room in one of the leading American IVF clinics, it is hard to resist the temptation. Beautiful picture albums on the coffee table show all of the babies conceived in this place, together with their beaming families. There is hope in the air. And a sign on the bulletin board offers the powerful message: You Never Fail until You Stop Trying.

A social worker at another IVF center criticized this kind of pressure:

> It is a rare bird, the infertility specialist who will say to couples, "Why don't you stop? Why don't you just put it in

park?" Even to take a break. It's very hard for couples to give themselves permission to say, "I have done enough." We need to really help people, when they need to say enough is enough, to be able to do that.

Stopping is particularly difficult for those couples who have achieved a pregnancy that ended in miscarriage or ectopic pregnancy. They have tasted success; for them IVF worked, at least for a while. After years of trying to get pregnant, they have finally done it, and they celebrate their accomplishment. The clinic celebrates with them, counting them as a success. As one program director said:

> It took us more than fifteen transfers to get our first pregnancy. If you've done fifteen with nothing, a pregnancy is a real shot in the arm, whether it results in a live birth or not. It's a shot in the arm for the medical team and for the other patients too, because they always want to know if you're having successes. And for some infertile people, even a failed pregnancy can be better than none at all.

Although a successful birth is still the exception, it does occur. One fortunate couple, whose daughter Carla is an IVF baby, are Sharon and Jerry.

Sharon had become pregnant quite unintentionally shortly after her marriage to Jerry, when she was in her twenties. They both knew they did not want another child right away after Alison was born, so they used birth control conscientiously, sure that they were superfertile. When they decided later to have another child, it never occurred to them that it might not work. Like many couples with secondary infertility, they were astonished to find out that what had been so easy six years earlier was now impossible. It was five long years until they finally had another daughter, Carla, conceived in a petri dish at a fertility clinic during their second attempt at IVF.

Sharon and Jerry described to us their experience with IVF. Sharon, still ecstatic, began:

> It's been a miracle. Carla was dropped from heaven and I feel so blessed. It's as if I've woken up from a nightmare. I am a new person—I am not infertile any more. I got pregnant and probably can again, if I want to. In fact, this turned my life around.
>
> Our problem, as it turned out, was damage to my tubes. I must have the most horrible tubes in fifty states. Even

when I first became pregnant with in vitro, I had an ectopic pregnancy. But that was hardly my first. During those five years we were trying to get pregnant, I actually conceived three times, but I had a miscarriage the first time, then two ectopic pregnancies and several operations to repair my tubes. The first ectopic was especially traumatic. I came pretty close to dying that time. I came within two hours of hemorrhaging to death. So much at once—my first major surgery, nearly dying, losing a pregnancy, and discovering how serious my infertility problem was all at once. I was pretty badly depressed after that.

Part of the difficulty in deciding on in vitro, even though our doctor said it was our only chance, was the fear of facing one more loss, one more failure. I had terrible feelings of guilt that my body was this damaged vessel that was not capable of letting life continue. It was difficult for me to think that I would be carrying around fertilized eggs that would die one more time. I didn't think I could stand any more dead babies.

The turning point for me came when a good friend said, "You know all those eggs in your ovaries are going to die when you do, and they are dying each month. Now you can take a risk that they'll live to ten or thirty cells, with the chance of becoming a human being, or not live at all." So I decided, OK, together me and my eggs will just take that risk of living to twenty cells or however far they get with the outside chance that one of them might actually continue—otherwise they'd die anyway.

Jerry continued the account:

We were actually very good candidates for the procedure, knowing that the tubes were our problem. I was more eager than Sharon to try it, thinking of it as a real challenge, almost an adventure into new scientific territory. Besides I just wasn't ready to consider adoption; I really wanted another child that was ours. We couldn't let the opportunity go by. One good thing about the in vitro was that it took the pressure off our marriage. I didn't have to perform according to the calendar, and lovemaking became more natural at that point.

Sharon interjected:

I think everybody goes into it believing it might work. Even though they tell you that the success rate is low, there's something very compelling about it. You get very much tied up into their system—you get to know the physicians and they get invested in you, and you see it work with other patients; so even if it doesn't work you try again. When you know that there's a chance out there, it's hard not to grab for it.

The whole system has such built-in hope, as you move from one stage to the next, that there's a lot of false optimism that gets built in. You know, all of a sudden, you've got follicles and you get a little excited about that. You go to the laparoscopy and they are able to view the eggs; you get real excited about that. As you move along the process, you get more and more hopeful, so that by the end there's only a very small part of you that's really ready for bad news.

Jerry remembered his feelings at the time of the final stage of the procedure:

I really believed that Sharon was pregnant after the embryos were transferred. I had even looked in the microscope to see the embryos, and when I said I wasn't sure what I was looking at, Sharon's response was, "What's the matter—don't you even recognize your own kid?" I was so sure that it would work since everything had gone perfectly up to that point. When we found out she was pregnant, we were elated and began to make plans for the birth. We were astonished at the grief and depression we felt when we realized she was having another ectopic.

Jerry and Sharon were both very involved in the in vitro procedure. They felt that in many ways it brought them together as a couple, since they were both so oriented to achieving pregnancy, and the procedure was something they could work on together. They were fortunate to have been referred to a clinic that had already been operating for two years, had had a number of successful births, and was less than two hours away from their home. They were able to get the Pergonal locally, and Jerry gave Sharon the shots at home. By the eighth day, however, she needed to be at the clinic early each morning for a week of ultrasounds and blood tests. She moved into a motel near the medical center. Sharon recalled that time:

Being there alone did not bother me. I looked upon it as kind of a nice vacation, and I knew that Jerry and our daughter Alison would be there for the weekend. There were several of us at the same motel, and we tended to spend a lot of time together. Most of the time it was very helpful, but occasionally the anxiety became contagious and that was the down side of it.

Jerry commented:

I think the hardest part for me was the waiting, waiting at home for Sharon to call while she was away to let me know if it was going okay. Then waiting outside the operating room during the laparoscopy—it brought back all the old anxieties of waiting outside during tubal surgery and ectopic pregnancy. I just felt so helpless then. When I saw her in recovery she was terribly nauseous and uncomfortable. And of course it was awful waiting for the results of the blood tests to see if she was pregnant.

Sharon continued their story:

After the embryos were transferred in one part of the hospital, they had to take me on a gurney to the hospital itself, because at that time you had to stay twenty-four hours. Well, it was the bumpiest ride I've ever been through and I thought, "This isn't good, I'm supposed to be perfectly still and I'm sure things are falling out." And then we had to wait for the elevator, and I was on an incline and I could feel things starting to drip out and I thought, "It's all over." I was very pessimistic at that point.

We were ecstatic when the test came back positive. But then I kept bleeding and having pain on one side and I called the doctor and told him this feels like an ectopic pregnancy again. They discovered I was right, and they removed the fallopian tube. I was so scared by this experience that I asked them to please cauterize the other tube way down at the base. These tubes were no friends of mine.

At that point I was hopeful because before I hadn't been able to part with my tubes, they were my only chance. Now that I got pregnant once, I figured I could do it again. They could take my tubes—I didn't need them any more. I think that knowing I could get pregnant, that it worked, made it easier for me to accept the loss. Instead of feeling helpless, I could go on. Also, I'm a somewhat religious person, and I just felt that if God wanted this for me it would be. If not, then that was His will and I could accept what would happen. That was very helpful and kind of got me through it.

The hardest part was probably the emotional aspect of it. I was very psyched for this the second time. I felt very positive about it, knowing that if I could just get pregnant and have it in the right place, I would be on my way. I had decided I would do this as often as necessary to get pregnant, no matter how long it took. And yet I kept trying to tell myself that it might not work, the success rate wasn't good, because I was so afraid of another disappointment. And then the embryo that was to be Carla was transferred to me on Mother's Day—what a good omen!

I knew it wasn't over when that pregnancy was confirmed. I just didn't believe it was going to last, that I could be so lucky. All through the pregnancy I kept waiting for something to happen, for it to be taken away from me. But I also figured that if one embryo survived out of the six that were transferred, this must be a strong and healthy one.

I think I had the same concerns for her that I would have had if I had conceived her naturally. It was a relief when she was born to see that she was a very healthy baby. Now when I look at her, I don't even think about all we went through to get her. She's just Carla, a very special child.

The Risks of IVF

Certainly one concern for couples is the risks of the procedure, both for the woman and for the potential baby. IVF pregnancies are more likely to end in ectopic pregnancy, miscarriage, or premature birth. It has been difficult, however, to assess the significance of the high rates of loss, because the women involved may be at a higher risk of experiencing these losses than other women by virtue of their age and infertility history.[12]

There is little evidence available about the risks involved in taking fertility drugs, and physicians claim that they have been proven safe over many years of use. Yet one IVF center's consent form warns of the rare possibility of kidney failure and death from Pergonal. Serious questions have also been raised about the long-term effects of repeated ultrasounds, although again the evidence is inconclusive.[13] Doctors usually minimize the risks, and patients usually do not ask. Many say they will do whatever is necessary and do not consider the possible side effects. As one nurse at an IVF clinic said:

Patients are not frightened about what is going to happen to their bodies. It's amazing, if you told them we'll have to tie your arms and legs down or whatever it is, they are willing to go through it.

Probably the greatest risk of the IVF procedure is a laparoscopy, since any use of general anesthesia carries the risk of complications and (rarely) of death. Many women reported that the nausea after the anesthesia was the most unpleasant part of the whole procedure. A more recently developed method of egg retrieval, known as ultrasound-guided aspiration, is making it possible to avoid laparoscopy in many cases. A thin needle is inserted into the ovary either through the vagina or by way of the bladder. Using ultrasound to visualize the eggs, the physician can remove them through the needle without a general anesthetic, at considerable savings of money and stress. Some programs offer this method as an office procedure. The major disadvantage so far has been the smaller number of eggs that can be obtained, thus possibly reducing the likelihood of pregnancy.[14]

No evidence from animals or humans suggests that babies conceived by IVF are at any greater risk of birth defects or other problems than babies conceived naturally. Yet most scientists agree that there is the theoretical potential for abnormalities as a result of the procedure. It is too early to be sure, since the numbers are still small and most of the children too young for definitive assessment.[15]

One risk that is widely acknowledged is that of multiple births. Twins, triplets, quadruplets are all much more common with IVF. They occur in 10 to 20 percent of pregnancies when more than one embryo is transferred. This occurrence has presented a serious dilemma: On the one hand, the more embryos transferred, the better the chances for a pregnancy. Yet multiple births increase the dangers for the mother and babies and may present overwhelming problems of parenting.[16]

One woman who underwent IVF dismissed the problem: "For a woman who's infertile, multiple births are multiple blessings." However, another couple that had tried for a long time to have a baby realized they were unable to cope with the prospect of having four and decided to have an abortion instead when they learned that the wife was carrying quadruplets. This was a disaster for all concerned.

This kind of situation has led some physicians to prefer freezing some of the embryos until a later cycle rather than inserting all of them at once. Freezing also has the advantage of reducing the need for renewed drug therapy and surgery on each attempt. But freezing embryos is objectionable to many people and is still not well perfected.[17] To overcome the fears of many that frozen embryos will be experimented on or discarded, scientists are working on techniques for freezing eggs before fertilization instead. When this can be done easily, and the eggs can be thawed and fertilized in later cycles without damage, it is likely to be used widely.

◆　◆　◆　◆　◆

IVF may seem controversial to outsiders. The United States government, source of so much research support, refuses to fund IVF research, and many groups object to its use.[18] But to those involved with infertility, it is becoming an increasingly routine procedure. New techniques that avoid repeated surgery are likely to make the experience less traumatic. And the greater willingness of insurance companies to cover the cost is making it more accessible.

Scientists and fertility specialists applaud the opportunity they are giving couples to try to get pregnant. However, our initial questions remain. Is IVF a wonderful technology giving people another chance, or is it a false promise? Are couples really freely choosing to proceed, giving themselves another possibility, or does the sheer existence of IVF make it imperative that they try it?

We have seen many people excluded from trying IVF by the cost and by the rules of eligibility. We have seen the torment couples go through, the misrepresentation of success rates, the stress and grief, the reopening of old wounds thought healed. There is the possibility of more loss, the worry about risks and side effects, and a lack of support and follow-up.

Even so, couples told us, it was worth the try. Even if they did not have a baby, at least they had a chance. And when sometimes, blessedly, it worked, the happiness was unimaginable.

5
Surrogate
Motherhood

"How could you possibly give up your own baby for $10,000? What normal woman would ever do this?" These are the questions posed to surrogate mothers by others. There is hostility and bewilderment in the questioning.

A surrogate mother named Jan wrote a letter to the child she was carrying to explain her feelings about what she was doing.

> I'm sure you're wondering why I would do this. I have two children of my own who are very precious to me, and it's hard for me to envision going through life wanting children and not being able to have them. I felt that I could help your mom and dad out by doing this. ... Being pregnant with you has been very exciting, and something very special for myself. I felt very good ... but the best thing was the excitement I knew your mom and dad were experiencing. I've never thought of you as my child, but you hold a very special place in my heart.[1]

The majority of the American public is appalled by the idea that a woman could voluntarily agree to become pregnant (with the sperm of a man who is not her husband) and then give the baby to that man and his wife in exchange for $7,000, $10,000, or $12,000, and expenses. The "profamily" forces on the Right oppose the idea because of its potential for undermining the traditional family, one ruled by men whose wives' key roles are caretaker and babymaker. For example, they fear the possibility that women could hire surrogate mothers for convenience, to maintain their own careers. The feminist Left is just as fervently critical. Gena Corea, author of *The Mother Machine,* calls surrogates "breeders," women whose bodies are being used to produce children for men. Lawyers and ethicists debate whether this is baby selling or not, and physician organizations have expressed serious reservations about the ethics and risks of surrogate motherhood.[2]

Opinion surveys on alternatives for having babies show surrogate mothering to be at the very bottom of everyone's list.[3] Many people simply do not understand what it is all about and assume that a man must sleep with the surrogate for her to become pregnant. The idea of receiving money for a baby is discomforting, perhaps even more so because it is a woman taking payment for something she's supposed to do for free, as part of her role in life.

What does this practice say about "maternal instinct"? Must a woman be abnormal or unnatural to get involved in such a project? Ironically most of the women who serve as surrogates are fairly conventional in their life-styles. They are not radicals or prostitutes, but wives and mothers who love being pregnant and think that having children is extremely important.

The term *surrogate mother* is used here because it is the most recognized name for women who have babies for others. It is misleading, however, perhaps intentionally so, since the term *surrogate* usually refers to a substitute for the real thing. At the time of the birth, the surrogate mother is actually the real mother, a mother who has agreed to give up her child to its father and his wife.[4]

Who uses surrogate programs? Mostly affluent couples with a fertile husband and an infertile wife, for whom other treatments have failed and adoption is unavailable or unacceptable. The woman may have a genetic disease that she does not want to transmit or a medical condition that precludes pregnancy.

At least one program has also accepted single men who want to father children. A very unusual case occurred in this program. A man preparing for a sex change operation wanted to inseminate a surrogate mother so that he would be the father of the child as well as its mother after his operation. However, due to the hormone treatments he was receiving, he had become infertile. These situations are still very much the exception. It is the exception, however, that confirms for many people that such programs are bizarre.

All this controversy did not deter Sarah, a thirty-one-year-old secretary who had a baby for Alex and Lisa. She feels good about what she did, sure that it was right:

> I knew how I would feel if I didn't have my children. I mean my children are my whole life. I just can't imagine not having them.
>
> My best friend couldn't get pregnant, and yet it was so easy for me. I know the kind of anguish she went through. I couldn't help her, but I felt a need inside me to help someone else. Thank God I'm healthy enough to do it.
>
> I loved being pregnant. I liked the attention, but my family is complete. My husband and I don't want any more children for ourselves—he had a vasectomy a few years ago. At first the money made it attractive too, but after I got pregnant and started to feel so close to Lisa, it didn't seem very important any more. I was not even sure I'd be able to accept the money.
>
> I like the idea of doing something unique. But basically I'm just a normal person, not someone who is out for money. But I'm not some kind of angel either. I'm just a normal working-class woman who does it because I like being pregnant and I like giving other people the happiness that my kids have given me.

It has been a decade since attorney Noel Keane started the first surrogate program in Michigan. Since then, more than twenty programs have started in other states, and more than five hundred babies have been born to surrogate mothers.[5] In very few of these cases (five that we are aware of) has the surrogate mother changed her mind and kept the baby.

How do women who want to be surrogates and couples who want a baby find each other? Sometimes a couple recruits a woman through personal networks or advertisements. Occasionally, a family member—a sister or a cousin—offers to carry a baby for her infertile relative. Most often, however, they are brought together by "matchmakers"—attorneys, physicians, psychologists, former surrogate mothers and others—who have started surrogate programs.

Alex and Lisa were at first skeptical about trying a surrogate program. They had been through a miscarriage, an ectopic pregnancy, tubal surgery, and three failed attempts of IVF (in vitro fertilization). They were on an adoption list but discouraged by the years they would still have to wait. Lisa described how hard it was to decide:

> I knew how important it was for Alex to have his own baby and I felt guilty that I couldn't provide that for him. I wanted one too, but I had finally begun to accept the reality that I would never give birth to my own baby. I saw a TV program about surrogates but couldn't handle the idea at the time. I got depressed just thinking about it. The idea of giving up on my own body and looking at someone else's and visualizing that person being the biological parent of my child was too painful for me.
>
> A year later we still didn't have a baby, and the thought of a surrogate mother began to seem more like a possibility. I showed Alex an article about it and was surprised at how enthusiastic he was. I was willing to talk to the attorney at least and find out more about it.

Alex saw the advantages of a surrogate program right away:

> I figured we'd have more control with a surrogate than with adoption, where somebody arbitrarily thinks this baby will fit well with this couple. I liked the idea that both of us would be there at the start of creating a baby. The child would know that he or she was created not by accident but out of love and a commitment to nurture that child for the rest of our lives. And of course at least we knew that the baby would have half of our genes.

Screening Couples and Surrogates

After finally deciding to contact a surrogate program, Lisa and Alex were worried about being accepted. As it turned out, there was no screening process whatsoever. The lawyer told them he accepted all couples who could pay. He explained his reasoning in an interview with us:

> It is his child and he has a constitutional right to do this. We have no basis for screening the couple. They've been through enough torture already. If they were able to conceive on their own, no one would ask them "How many windows do you have facing the lawn?" or "How much money did you earn?" the way people who want to adopt are questioned.

Different programs vary greatly in their philosophies regarding the selection of couples. Three programs described here—referred to as the East Coast, Midwest, and California programs—represent some of the variations that can be found. For example, some programs, such as the East Coast one, require that couples be married and childless and have a documented fertility problem. Otherwise they have no screening of applicants. The Midwest program, on the other hand, accepts everyone who applies. They may see a psychiatrist, but only if they request it.

In contrast, the California program has very different policies. The psychologist who interviews all the couples who come to the program explained to us that acceptance is far from automatic:

> What I screen them for is appropriateness for a surrogate mother program, not appropriateness for parenthood. I'm not like an adoption agency. I want to know if they can handle our philosophy and how we work. I say to them, "Let me help you decide if this is the way that's best for you."
>
> They're very anxious for a child and willing to be flexible. But occasionally we have a couple who are not ready for a surrogate. They have to come to terms with the third party in a very physical way—the woman may be in the delivery room or at Lamaze classes, and she'll be talking to the surrogate periodically. If a woman's infertility is not resolved to the point where she can handle being with the woman who's carrying her husband's child, it's going to be painful.

The three programs also have conflicting ideas about how to select the women to be surrogate mothers. All have some kind of screening by a psychologist or psychiatrist, but with very different intentions. The psychiatrist who sees applicants to the Midwest program feels strongly that all applicants should be screened. But he also believes that if he finds a woman who wants to be a surrogate competent to make an informed decision, she has a right to be one. He said:

> I function by helping surrogates to screen themselves. I explain all the possible risks, and then the responsibility to decide is up to them. Professionals have no way to predict who will be OK. Even if we did know, our job should be to help them decide, not to be paternalistic and decide for them. What I advise is, "If you're not sure, don't do it. It's

forever; this is one of the most important decisions of your life."

He has interviewed well over five hundred applicants and has yet to turn one down, but a large proportion have dropped out on their own.

Surrogates are accepted in the Midwest program whether they are single, married, gay, have children, or not. The first surrogate in this program was an unmarried virgin, the infertile couple's friend who volunteered to have their baby. The program directors prefer, however, that surrogates have children already. They used to think it was better if the women were single or divorced, anticipating possible complications from a husband. Now they believe that having a husband may be valuable for support. It also may be easier for the surrogate to give up a baby because it is not her husband's.

The psychologist in the California program also screens the women who apply to become surrogate mothers. In contrast to the open-door policy of the Midwest program, he turns away at least two-thirds of the applicants. First, he requires that they already have children at home, explaining that a woman who has never had a pregnancy and delivery cannot really know what she is agreeing to. He also eliminates anyone who, in his judgment, would suffer from being a surrogate:

> I feel that it is my job to make sure that no one gets into this who would get hurt. Even though it's very difficult sometimes, I do tell women I think it's simply not in their best interest to be a surrogate, that they are so needy and that this isn't going to fulfill their need. We see ourselves as very protective.

Not surprisingly, in California there is a waiting list of couples, while in the Midwest there are more surrogates than requests for them.

In California, the psychologist also sees husbands of potential surrogates to be sure that the women will have a supportive home environment. Once accepted, the surrogate is required, and the husband invited, to attend a monthly support group meeting. She is also in frequent contact with the psychologist.

The East Coast program has a different approach. Unlike the California program, which looks at the benefit or harm to the surrogate mothers, the East Coast program is concerned primarily with a woman's emotional ability to give away a child. According to the psychologist who screens all their applicants, he looks for women who are strong willed and reliable, and he accepts fewer than half of those who apply.

The Relationship between Surrogate Mother and Couple

Lisa and Alex were not aware of all these differences when they picked a surrogate program. They simply went to one located near their home. They were pleased, however, that the lawyer said they could meet Sarah before deciding if they wanted her to have a baby for them. Alex described what they were looking for:

> We wanted a nice normal human being who has above average intelligence. We wanted her to be emotionally stable, kind of a solid person. We thought it was important for her to be healthy and loving so that we would be able to communicate that to the child.

In a number of programs, the couple picks a woman from pictures in a book that includes details of the surrogates' history and motivations. Some come to the office to meet several women. Sometimes, if they request it, the director suggests a particular woman for a couple and then has them make the decision. All three people involved have to agree with the choice.

At the East Coast program, the attorney makes the match strictly according to the couple's place on the waiting list. When a surrogate becomes available, he sends a description and photograph of her and her children to the first couple on the list. If possible, two such profiles are sent, and the couple makes the decision.

In contrast to programs where the couples select among a number of women, the psychologist in the California program decides on every match. She sends to the couple and to the potential surrogate information about each other; if they are pleased with what they see, they must meet together with the program staff. Each party has a chance to veto the match, but as the psychologist says, "If I've done my job, it shouldn't happen, and it rarely does."

The most important difference among program staff is their attitude toward the relationship between surrogate mother and couple. Some programs leave that decision up to the parties involved. Other programs take definite, but opposite, stands on this issue. In California, for example, a meeting is required and a relationship encouraged, while in the East Coast program, complete anonymity is the rule.

The psychologist for the California program explained why she and her colleagues feel so strongly about openness:

> If the couple really doesn't want to meet the surrogate or they want to make sure she doesn't know where they are or what their last name is, it's not going to work. The surrogate is going to feel she's not being appreciated or that they don't trust her, or that they're still ashamed of this. And separation from the baby will be much harder. It works for us because she cannot imagine hurting this couple whom she knows and likes so much.

The East Coast program takes the opposite view. The program's directors feel strongly that, if a relationship were allowed to develop, the surrogate would have a harder time detaching herself from the couple and the child. They worry that she might refuse to be inseminated by an unattractive man, or that she would say, "This guy looks like Burt Reynolds, how can I give up Burt Reynolds's baby?" Therefore, couples and surrogates never meet and never learn each other's names or addresses. All communication is through the attorney's office.

So many differences; yet the key people in each program are confident that their way works best. They all base their policies on what they believe to be psychologically healthy and most efficient. Until follow-up studies are carried out, however, we cannot know which will prove to be the best for surrogate mothers, for couples, and especially for the children.

Generally, the couples seem to be more interested in anonymity than the surrogates. They feel uncertain about what part a known surrogate mother should continue to play in their lives. They worry about a meeting leading to problems. One woman explained:

> Suppose she didn't like my husband's glasses, or his freckles. Considering the enormity of what she's doing, something trivial like that could set her off. We just didn't want to take the risk. We had all the information we needed about her and the pregnancy from the lawyer.

Some surrogates fear that if they get to know the couple, it will be hard to separate from them as well as from the baby. They prefer a more "businesslike" arrangement, with no contact or information.

A more common situation is that of the woman who agrees to have a baby for an anonymous couple and then regrets the lack of contact. We heard stories, for example, of women who requested the baby's picture and received no response. One surrogate recalled:

> Once I was pregnant, I started having a lot of thoughts about the couple, wondering what kind of people I was going to be giving this baby to. I knew I could never meet them, and that began to bother me. I just hope that when the baby's older they'll tell her about me and let her come to see me if she wants to.

Occasionally both parties are obsessed with secrecy. Surrogates tell everyone that the baby died, and infertile wives pretend to be pregnant for nine months. We do not know the consequences of these behaviors, but we strongly suspect that such deception will be harmful to the people involved.

An Experience with Surrogate Mothering

Lisa, Alex, and Sarah discovered that it was very valuable for them to know each other. Eventually they forged strong bonds of commitment and friendship. Their relationship was stronger than most between surrogates and couples because they all wanted it that way. Although their story is unusual because of the closeness they developed, their experiences and feelings are shared by many others who became involved in surrogate programs.

The relationship began with a difficult introduction in the dark-leather conference room of a law firm. Sarah remembered that day vividly:

> The meeting was very awkward at first because you're going in feeling, "I really want to do this and I really want to please them." They're going in and they want to show that they really would be good parents and want a surrogate to have a baby for them. After about five or six minutes

of awkwardness, we started to chat and then we even got
into talking about things like my period and her uterus and
ovaries. It was odd talking about intimate subjects to
people you just met. It was important to me that they have
a very religious sense, that they believe in God, and not be
cold people. They were wonderful, and I knew by the end
of that meeting that I wanted to be the mother of their
baby. When they said they were sure they wanted me to be
their surrogate, I was so thrilled—I felt an immediate bond
with them.

As friendly as this threesome felt, they were uncomfortable
about starting the inseminations. Sarah had started charting her
temperature every day, and when she thought she was about to
ovulate, she called the program's physician. He arranged for her
and Alex to come in the next afternoon. Sarah described what
happened then:

It was all very odd. Lisa came with him and she and I are
sitting there chatting in the waiting room while Alex goes
in the bathroom. He comes out with the stuff and then I go
in the other room to have it inseminated. Then we all leave
on the elevator together just like this is an everyday
occurrence.

When I got home it hit me all of a sudden that I had
another man's sperm inside me and I might get pregnant by
him. It felt really creepy for a few minutes, but then it
passed. When I got my period that month, I was really
disappointed that it hadn't worked and eager to try again.

The second month Alex wasn't able to get here at the
right time, and Lisa decided to bring the sample by plane,
since they live four hours away by car. I always laugh when
I picture her running through the airport with her little
lunch bag. She didn't want it to go through the X rays, and
the security people asked, "What's this?" She tried to be
casual—"Oh, it's sperm," and they let her through.

When it took that time I was ecstatic. I called the
lawyer's office right away to tell him. I had a bouquet of
balloons sent to Lisa and Alex to let them know I was so
happy being pregnant. I proudly told everybody around me
that I was pregnant. I told my two sons, who were three
and a half and seven at the time, that I was having a baby for
Alex and Lisa. I explained to them that Lisa's tummy didn't
work and I would be carrying this baby for them. When I
referred to the baby, I would always says Lisa and Alex's

baby. They didn't have any problems with it. My son even told his class at school, "Guess what—my mommy's pregnant and we are not keeping the baby."

My sister and parents accepted it very easily. The only family member that gave me a hard time was my husband's aunt—she is a very staunch Catholic. She said, "God will punish you for this." "Aunt Rita," I said, "I find it hard to believe that God would punish me for giving so much love and happiness to someone else. I am happy with myself and feel good about what I am doing."

My pregnancy was easy—I wasn't tired or sick. But suddenly this all changed. During my tenth week I saw some blood. It hit me in the face like a thunderbolt that I could lose this baby. A few days later, blood started pouring out and I had excruciating labor pains—I thought I was really dying. However, I only worried about what I was going to tell Lisa and Alex. What a failure I was! Would they give up on me?

Sarah seemed to have had a strong need for Lisa and Alex's approval. She was more concerned about them than about the trauma her own body was going through. This is not unusual; some women become surrogates because of the positive attention they receive from the couple as well as from the professionals who run the program.

Fearful of rejection, Sarah wrote a letter to Lisa and Alex explaining how badly she felt. She said she felt she was their last hope and had let them down. She hoped they would want to try again with her.

Lisa and Alex were discouraged by the miscarriage and began to wonder if they just were not meant to have a baby. But Sarah's determination infused them with new hope. They called Sarah and told her they felt lucky to have her and that they wanted to continue as soon as she was ready.

After the miscarriage, Lisa and Alex visited Sarah's home and met her family for the first time. Each meeting brought them closer together, and Sarah's husband Mike became more involved as well. He commented:

After they left, I talked to Sarah that night and told her, "That couple deserves to have a baby." Just because the woman he chose to marry cannot have children, that does not negate his right to have a child. And because I was lucky enough to marry someone who can have children, does that give me more of a right to have them? I just can't believe that. I think what Sarah's doing is fantastic—I'm really proud of her.

By the time they started trying again, Lisa felt they could do without the physician. After all, insemination is a simple procedure, one that can be accomplished with a store-bought syringe, and she wanted her baby conceived in a more personal environment. Lisa replied:

We invited her to our house for a few days and I helped her do it several times. She and I would just lay on my bed and put up our feet together and just talk for an hour. It's so special that our baby was actually conceived in our own bed.

Lisa and Alex almost held their breaths until the second pregnancy had progressed beyond the first trimester. Even then they were still very tense. We talked to Lisa halfway through the pregnancy:

I'm excited, but nervous too. There's just been so much suppressed feeling for so long and we're trying to suppress it for another four or five months—it's hard. I think the uneasiness is irrational, it's nothing specific. But just to have a baby live, you know—I just sort of hold it in and try to stay very busy.

I'm really very glad though that the baby's in her uterus and not mine. It would be dead if it were in my body, and so there's really a feeling of relief and trusting her body over mine.

We've already been there for a couple of prenatal visits. Hearing the heart beat, seeing the baby on ultrasound—I can't tell you how thrilling this has been. We even framed the ultrasound picture and hung it by our bed so we could see it whenever we wanted to. Sarah is incredible—she sent us Mother's Day and Father's Day cards and a tape of the baby's heart beat. We played it so many times the tape wore out. I talk to her at least once a week to find out how she's doing. It keeps me feeling very connected to the pregnancy.

Alex did not have the frequent contact with Sarah. He dealt with his anxiety by trying to be more detached. It didn't help that he was still uncomfortable with the whole idea. Alex described his feelings:

> I still would rather it be Lisa carrying my baby, and sometimes I get angry at Sarah for not being Lisa, for being able to do what my own wife cannot. I know that's not fair, but I can't help how I feel. In some ways it would have been easier if we didn't meet her and know what a wonderful human being she is. It's more difficult than just renting a womb, so to speak. And she needs a lot of attention from us—if Lisa doesn't call one week, Sarah starts to wonder what's going on.

Sarah did want the attention and the reassurance she gained from those visits and calls. She relied on Lisa to help her through the difficult times when she was feeling ambivalent or uncertain. Sarah recalled:

> Whenever I had any maternal feelings toward the baby, like when it first started to move, I would call up Lisa and talk it through with her. That way I just transferred those feelings to Lisa. I never felt this was my baby. I tacked a picture of Lisa and Alex on my refrigerator so that all of us could keep in mind that I was doing this for them. If I ever thought about keeping the baby, all I'd have to do is look at that picture and think what they've been through.
>
> Not everyone was as lucky as me, having Lisa to talk to. I've talked to other women who are having a very hard time. I think support groups should be required for us, to help handle the criticism for one thing. Also, being able to deal with the fact that some day you're going to have a child in your arms and you are going to hand that child over to somebody else. You can gear yourself up for the nine months, but when it comes you're still going to have a difficult time.

Lisa moved into Sarah and Mike's house two weeks before the due date, wanting to make sure she was there for the baby's arrival. She felt very close to Sarah's family during that time.

Everyone worried about how the hospital staff would react to their situation. Would they allow Lisa into the delivery room? Would she be able to hold the baby? As it turned out, with some help from the program's physician, the labor nurses reluctantly agreed to go along. Sarah remembers the delivery vividly:

When I started pushing, Lisa was pushing with me. There were tears in her eyes when she saw the baby's head. I was so happy to see Lisa's pure joy. They handed the baby to me first and I looked at her for a minute and handed her to Lisa. Mike was by my side, and they let Alex come in to see his daughter. She was a beautiful 7 lb. 2 oz. healthy little girl. They named her Emily.

The nurse told me she had been on the labor floor twenty-five years and never in those twenty-five years had she ever witnessed such love in the delivery of a baby.

Alex had arrived at the hospital only a few minutes before Emily was born. He describes the incredible feelings of that moment:

It's a little hard to convey how wonderful that experience was. I was standing in the delivery room thinking, "What do I do now?" and there's this little pink prune squawking its head off and grabs onto my finger. There's a bonding that takes place—there's no lightning flash, but it's there. It's a moment that will be there forever for me. At that moment I had a daughter.

Sarah stayed in the hospital for three days. Lisa and Alex were staying at her house, but they spent every waking moment at the hospital, sharing in the care of the baby. This was not an easy time for Sarah, as she recalls:

In the hospital the second night the baby was in the room with me, and I looked down at her sweet face and thought she looked just like me. I immediately called Lisa to talk to her about how well her baby was doing and my feeling about the baby. As I was talking the baby fell asleep and I felt better.

Lisa and Alex stayed at our house one more night after I came home from the hospital. That night I had a difficult experience. The baby was in Lisa and Alex's room and I could hear her screaming. They were trying to calm her, but just like any new parents, they werent' sure what to do. I felt torn between wanting to help the baby and feeling that it was important to let them handle her themselves.

The hardest part was saying good-bye to them the next day. I had a much harder time saying good-bye to Lisa than to the baby because I had such an intensely close relationship with her. Even though I knew our relationship would continue, it would be different. That good-bye really caught me off guard because I hadn't expected it.

After they left, it was like that feeling I have the day after Christmas. The parties are over, the presents have been opened, and all the anticipation, all the fun, is over. All that is left are empty boxes and torn wrapping paper. Mike put his arm around me and told me how wonderful he thought I was, and how much he loved me. It really helped having his support. One of the things that was hard for both of us was the fact that the baby was a girl and we have two sons. If it had been a boy I think it would have been much easier.

Lisa was simply overwhelmed by all that had happened. She remembers:

> I was just so grateful to Sarah, and ecstatic to finally have our baby. I told Sarah she had made it possible for us to have the family we never thought we could have, and to experience a pregnancy as much as we ever could. There were no words to tell her how happy she had made us, but I'm sure she understood. I worried about her though, I hoped she would be OK.

During the first few weeks after Emily's birth, Sarah and Lisa talked on the phone often. They needed to reassure each other that everything was all right. Sarah said:

> I probably have my highest euphoria when I am talking to Lisa. When I hear her talking to Emily or she's drinking her bottle while Lisa's talking to me, I think, she just sounds like a really different person than what she did when I met her. She sounds very content now, like she is complete. That is the biggest gift that she could have given me, just letting me hear her be happy like that.

One month later, Sarah was in court, declaring before a judge her intention to relinquish all rights to the baby. She knew that up until that time she could change her mind. But whenever she was tempted to do so, she thought about how ecstatic Alex and Lisa were and realized she could never break their hearts. She had taken on an important job, had done it well, and had gained valuable friends. She knew that she would be part of their lives in some way, that she could always know how the child was doing.

All of that made it hard for her to think about accepting the money that would arrive after the day in court. The payment is often a troubling subject for surrogate mothers, and they are sensitive to accusations of baby selling. The surrogates remind people, however, that they are giving the baby to his or her own father, not to strangers who have no connection. Some are reluctant to take the money, while for others the idea of a contractual obligation keeps them committed to relinquishing the baby. Sarah said:

It was never my major motivation. If you think about it, $10,000 isn't a lot of money for all of the inconvenience and discomfort of the inseminations and pregnancy and birth. At least I didn't have to abstain from sex with my husband during the inseminations like most of the other women. We were grateful for that vasectomy. Even so, it was a year out of my life.

Mike and I had decided that we couldn't take any money from Alex and Lisa. Yet they insisted, telling me I deserved it, that there is no way that any amount of money they could give me would ever be enough to reward me for what I had done for them. Lisa made me feel comfortable about taking the money, just as I had made her feel comfortable about taking the child when she was worrying so much about taking her from me. There was something else—much more important than the money. The day we signed the papers, Lisa gave me a string of pearls. I had no idea it was coming, and I wear them all the time.

Sarah used the money to go back to school and start a new career. She felt she had given a precious gift to Alex and Lisa and had received in turn a new direction for her own life, a new sense of confidence and specialness.

Obviously not many couples can afford the $25,000 to $30,000 an average surrogate program costs, including legal, medical, and counseling fees as well as expenses and the fee for the surrogate. Those who can, however, are happy to pay it. A private adoption, or five or six IVF attempts, would cost as much. As Alex said:

I think the surrogate deserves a larger fee for everything she's done. There's so much else involved for them. For us, it wasn't easy to come up with such a big amount. Let me put it this way—I could have bought one helluva Porsche. But then, on the other hand, if I had bought a Porsche, that's all I'd have, and there's no comparison to having Emily.

Problems with Surrogate Mothering

The experience we have described is in many ways unusual. Most surrogates and couples do not develop such a close relationship. Some surrogates want this kind of relationship, or at least more contact than they have, but they do not know how to make it happen. The program may not allow it, or the couple may not want it. Other surrogates prefer to think about what they are doing as more like a job and manage to maintain a certain detachment from the whole process. Program psychologists are still surprised by the number of women who do not seek any support or any information about the couple and the baby.

Are surrogates fooling themselves by treating surrogate motherhood like a temporary job? Are they rationalizing away bothersome emotions? Or are these simply unique women for whom being a surrogate mother brings sufficient rewards (emotional or financial) to outweigh any discomfort or pain? Some women even decide to become surrogates a second time; and this is true of both those who know the couple and those who do not.

There is no doubt that, for most women, being a surrogate mother is a difficult job. It requires tremendous commitment and has the potential to create serious problems. Uncertainty about the relationship to the couple, negative comments from others, and especially grief for the baby who is gone are all common.

Even the best-prepared surrogate mothers may have a difficult time adjusting, and they often find it hard to admit to needing help. One woman told us:

I think with surrogates there is this image you feel you must keep, that you are a "super surrogate" and you're not going to feel any feelings after the baby is born other than happiness for the couple because they finally got their child. But that's not true, because for nine months you carried this child. Every night you lay down in bed and you're laying on your side because the baby's there. And you get home and that baby is not there. It was not so much that I wanted to change my mind. It was just the feeling of emptiness because there wasn't a baby there when there should have been by all laws of nature.

A few programs provide support groups or individual counseling for the surrogate mothers while they are pregnant. Most women we interviewed felt there should be more, and that the feelings of loss should be addressed.

One woman who has become a resource for others in the program she was involved with explained some of the problems:

> Sometimes other surrogates call me because they are afraid to talk to the couple. Maybe they haven't met the couple and want to but aren't sure how to go about it. Or the couple does not want them to hold the baby at all in the hospital and they want to. I tell them, "Until you sign the papers giving up custody of that child, that child is yours. If you want to hold that baby, no one can stop you."
>
> Sometimes they want to find out more about the baby after it's born but can't. I think there is a need for more of a mediator between these people, and a way for them to talk to surrogates who've done it already.

Occasionally it is the couples who have to confront grief. An early case that received a lot of publicity was that of a surrogate mother who decided to keep her child even before the birth. The couple filed suit seeking custody. Before the trial it came out that the wife could not have children because she had had a sex change operation. Fearful that this information would work against them in court, the couple dropped the case a day before the trial and gave up any rights to the child.[6]

Another couple, who never had contact with the surrogate, flew six hundred miles to pick up their baby on the day his birth was scheduled to be induced. When they arrived, they were shocked to find out that the mother had never checked into the hospital. The wife recalled her traumatic experience:

> We called the person running the program to find out what happened. She seemed very upset on the phone and said the surrogate had gone to another hospital where no one would know about this baby's origin. And then she told us she would be right over to our hotel with the baby. As she handed the baby to us, she said we would not be able to keep him because the mother had changed her mind. She stood outside in the hall for twenty minutes while we stood inside the room too stunned to talk or look at each other. We just watched our little baby boy whom we would probably never see again. Then she knocked on the door, and like robots we handed her back the baby. There we were in that strange room far from home, surrounded by all the baby clothes and diapers we brought with us.

> We signed a legal document that said we weren't sure
> who the biological father was and gave up all our rights and
> responsibilities and got our money back. We didn't sue
> because we were sure we wouldn't have a chance of getting
> him. Who would take a nursing baby from his mother?

This couple was in a program in the Midwest where the surrogate and couple are not allowed to meet. Although they ex-
changed letters through the program office, the wife feels the
main reason the surrogate mother kept the baby was because of
this policy. She said:

> We were anonymous to her, we weren't real people. She
> needed emotional support and wasn't getting it from the
> program. We should have been there to give it to her.
> Instead, we were strangers that she was supposed to give
> her baby to. *We* knew we would be good parents, but she
> had no way to know that.

This woman was sure that no court would award her the
child. Yet, in a complicated and dramatic New Jersey case which
has brought a great deal of attention to surrogate mothering, one
genetic father did challenge in court the surrogate mother's decision to keep the child. The mother, Mary Beth Whitehead, had
given the baby to the father, William Stern, and his wife, but a
few days later she asked to have the child back for a week. When
the week elapsed and Whitehead did not return, police tried to
seize the infant. Whitehead fled the state with the baby but was
discovered several months later by private detectives. At the
time of this writing, "Baby M" has been awarded to the Sterns
and the surrogate contract decisively upheld. Whitehead is ap-
pealing the decision, which terminates a surrogate's right to
change her mind from the moment she conceives. This case will
have a major influence on the future of surrogate programs. It
has certainly demonstrated that surrogate motherhood can turn
into tragedy for all involved, especially for the birth mother.[7]

Until this case, the legal status of surrogate mothering has
been untested and therefore unclear. Most states have laws
against black market adoption, in which the birth mother is paid
by the adoptive couple. Many also have ruled, in response to
AID, that the man whose sperm is used to inseminate a woman
is not legally the father. In addition, a number of legislators have
introduced bills to regulate surrogate mothering.[8]

Despite all of the potential problems, each program has so far managed to find legal ways to accomplish its goals. According to one program director, "We do not confront laws any more; we find out procedurally what's the easiest position to take. We find out where the least resistance is in order to complete this." Many attorneys associated with surrogate programs look for states that have stepparent adoption statutes. Since the father's name is already on the birth certificate, and he is recognized in some states as the legal father, his wife can adopt the child as a stepparent.

Sarah maintains that her experience, at least, was a positive one, although she longs for the baby and wonders sometimes what life would be like if Emily were with her:

> When I think back about the whole experience, I really feel good about myself and what I did for them. I wear my pearls almost all the time and I talk to Lisa pretty often. However, as time goes by, Lisa calls less often, and I feel disappointed. They invited all of us to come visit them on Emily's first birthday. I was glad to see her Mom and Dad so happy and they are really good parents to Emily. But it was a shock to see Emily. She looks so much like me. Seeing her reminded me how much I had wanted my own baby girl.
>
> Lisa and Alex asked me if I would think about having a brother or sister for Emily. I told them I didn't think I could do it again.
>
> Being with them, it felt just like an extended family. It was hard to leave though. I knew it would probably be a long time until I saw Emily again.

6
Ovum Transfer

In January 1984, the first baby to have been carried by two mothers was born. This young boy is the product of an unusual partnership of medical researchers, financiers, and a livestock breeder. He was conceived inside of one woman who had been inseminated with the sperm of the other woman's husband. Five days after conception, the tiny embryo was removed without surgery and transplanted into the uterus of the second woman. This woman, who was infertile, then carried the baby to term and gave birth to him. This birth, and that of a girl born several months later, represent the first successes of a method called ovum transfer (OT). A third baby was born in Milan, Italy, in 1986.

Although OT is a relatively new procedure for humans, it has been widely used in the cattle industry for some time to increase the number of offspring of genetically superior cows. These high-quality cows are inseminated with the sperm of prize bulls. Their embryos are then removed, to be carried by more common cattle, so that the superior cow can be inseminated again very quickly.[1]

Richard Seed, a consultant to the livestock industry, with his physician brother Randolph, began a corporation in 1978 named Fertility and Genetics Research (FGR). Its purpose has been to apply ovum transfer to humans. A grant to Drs. John Buster, John Marshall, and colleagues at Harbor-UCLA Medical Center made it possible to carry out the first experimental phase in 1983 and 1984.

Once the "research phase" was completed, FGR sought financing to expand its operations. Since December 1985 the company's stock has been traded over the counter under the symbol "BABYU." The company is currently involved in creating OT clinics in joint ventures with hospitals and physician groups in California, Chicago, and other major population areas in Europe and the United States.

The second phase of OT started in the fall of 1986 in Long Beach, California, at a private medical center. Ultimately, according to James Twerdahl, a former electronics executive who is president of FGR, the intention is to have thirty to fifty such OT centers in North America. Once the first clinics prove successful, FGR plans to develop new ones in almost every metropolitan area in the United States, all under the corporation's control.

The developers of this new method call it *ovum transfer*, even though it is a five-day-old embryo that they transfer. The avoidance of the term *embryo transfer* in the OT program appears to be designed to allay public worries about scientists playing with embryos. Dr. John Buster, the professor of obstetrics and gynecology who directed the original OT research, talked about the careful selection of a name for the program:

> We chose the word *ovum* because, in 1980 when we prepared the protocol, we were concerned that there would be people parading with signs outside that we were transplanting things with arms and legs and eyes that we called an embryo.

The method has actually been given a number of names by different authors, including *surrogate embryo transfer*, *artificial embryonation*, and *prenatal adoption*. We refer to it as OT because it is likely that the name used by its developers will be most widely recognized. It also avoids confusion with IVF programs' common use of the term *embryo transfer* to refer to the insertion of fertilized eggs into the mother's uterus after two days of growing in a petri dish.

Ovum transfer could potentially create major changes in the process of reproduction which could affect fertile as well as infertile woman. First, the procedure offers infertile women a nonsurgical alternative to IVF that, if successful, would produce children who are related genetically to their husbands but not to themselves. Second, the OT program is important because its commercialization of infertility treatment departs from the usual medical approach. In addition to being financed by investors buying shares through the stock exchange, the program also operates out of profit-making clinics and FGR is seeking to patent the entire procedure. Third, OT may soon be the basis for diagnosing the genetic makeup and potential health problems of all embryos very early in their development.[2]

Ovum Transfer as an Infertility Treatment

The most obvious candidates for OT are women who cannot produce their own eggs. They may have had their ovaries removed or experienced premature menopause. In addition, women who are not infertile but do not want to take the chance of passing a genetic disease to their children might welcome the chance to be pregnant by carrying another woman's egg fertilized by their own husbands' sperm.[3]

FGR lists many such conditions that would bring couples to OT, but the initial research focused on, and was only successful with, women who had tubal problems. Only the OT baby born in Milan in 1986 had a mother without ovaries. The mothers of the first two OT babies born in California had normal ovaries but scarred fallopian tubes. In fact, the owners of FGR expect a major portion of their customers to come from the growing ranks of women, like these, who may have tried other methods such as IVF and failed. As FGR president Twerdahl told us:

> If a couple can afford it and they have their own sperm and eggs, we presume they would prefer IVF. But perhaps they can no longer afford IVF or they failed at IVF a couple of times. Perhaps the patient can't tolerate surgery and anesthesia anymore, whether she can't physically or psychologically. Then ovum transfer becomes a method for them.

Selecting Donors and Couples

In 1981, the ovum transfer program recruited its first donors by putting a small ad in the newspaper: "Help an infertile woman have a baby. Fertile women ages 20–35 willing to donate an egg. Similar to artificial insemination. No surgery required. Reasonable compensation." Of the four hundred women who answered the ad, many lost interest after their initial contact, and others were screened out. Only forty-six were finally accepted. Buster talked about the donors:

> To answer that ad was a pretty cavalier thing to do. . . . After screening out a bunch of people who weren't suitable, we were left with a few great ladies.

Those "few great ladies" were selected on the basis of psychological stability, medical suitability, proven fertility, and compliance. They and their husbands had been questioned at length to make sure they could handle the procedure and any possible side effects. Infertile couples who applied were also carefully screened to be sure they would fully cooperate with the program.[4] As Annette Brodsky, the psychologist in charge of screening, explained:

> You need people who are going to be stable enough to handle the fact that OT is a new procedure, that there might be publicity around it, that they won't get completely overwhelmed or thrown by the fact if something goes wrong. We didn't want them to be so invested in having a baby that, should prenatal testing reveal that the baby is deformed, they'd say they would want it anyway. Then the first baby in the project is deformed and the whole world stops wanting to think about it again.

In its current phase, in addition to putting ads in local newspapers to recruit donors, the OT program is now asking infertile couples to help find them. If a couple brings a friend or relative into the pool of donors, they will be given priority on the waiting list. Since there are 2,900 names on the list, this incentive puts a great deal of pressure on couples and their families.

The couples and donors who were finally selected to be part of the research phase never met each other, since the research team believed anonymity would be best. As they arrived at the barracks where inseminations and transfers took place, however, they wondered which of the other people who were coming and going would become so closely tied to them.

As a result of the donors' frustration at not knowing the results of their efforts, a major change was made in the policy of the program since the first experimental round. Now the directors intend to let the donors know if a woman becomes pregnant and has a baby with the donor's transferred eggs. In addition, contact between donors and couples will be possible for those who wish it. They will be asked to select one of three options: to know each other from the beginning, to have the possibility of meeting only when the child turns eighteen, or to have complete confidentiality unless the law changes this for the child's sake. Donors and couples will be matched according to which option they choose as well as according to physical characteristics.

Regardless of their choice, the recipient women who become pregnant will receive complete information about the donor's genetic and medical history as well as her life-style. By making this information available, the program directors hope to avoid some of the criticism that has been directed at AID and adoption for not allowing children to have information about their genetic heritage.

As the ovum transfer program grows nationally, donors and couples may be matched through a central computer. In a few collection centers around the country, "professional" donors will have numerous embryos washed out of them every month. These embryos can be frozen and shipped out to OT centers elsewhere in the country to waiting couples and their physicians.

The Procedure

The donors and the women recipients are matched for appearance and for their menstrual cycle. With large pools of both donors and infertile women, it should be possible to find women who match with each other. It is likely, however, that the number of donors will be small and that cycles will have to be synchronized with the use of hormones. It is also projected that donors will receive fertility drugs in order to create the possibility of more than one embryo per cycle.

After the matching is accomplished, the donor arrives at the clinic at the time of ovulation, to be inseminated by the sperm of the infertile woman's husband. The sperm have already been carefully examined for genetic information and the possibility of venereal disease. Five days after the insemination, the donor returns. With a specially designed catheter, about two ounces of fluid is flushed into her uterus. In a procedure called *lavage*, the fluid is then removed again through the catheter. If an embryo has been growing in the woman's uterus, it is unlikely to have attached itself yet to the uterine wall and therefore should emerge with the fluid. One woman who has been a donor described her experience:

> It's a simple procedure and doesn't take very long, about fifteen minutes from start to finish. You get undressed, get up on the table, put your feet in the stirrups. They use a speculum and then the catheter. There's a little bit of cramping; you feel a little tug for a second. It's pretty much like a regular exam.

The fluid taken from the donor's uterus is checked for embryos. If one is found, the recipient woman is called and the embryo is transferred, again by a catheter inserted through the cervix into the uterus. If everything goes as planned, the embryo that started in another woman's body will implant in the infertile woman's uterus and grow there normally.

Advantages and Disadvantages

Compared to IVF and many other treatments, OT is relatively simple and noninvasive. The embryo is conceived naturally in a woman's body instead of in a laboratory. At the time of the transfer, it has had approximately five days to develop in the donor, which should make it hardier than the two-day-old embryo transferred in IVF.

The major physical risks of OT are for the donor rather than for the couple. She is exposed to the possibility of infection through AID. She also risks remaining pregnant if the lavage process does not work. This has happened three times in OT research, and one of the donor women chose to have an abortion. The other two aborted spontaneously. Ectopic pregnancies are also a possibility, since the fluid could wash an embryo back up into the tubes.

To combat the risks of a retained pregnancy, donors will be given hormones in the form of a "morning-after" pill. Those who suffer an ectopic pregnancy may receive an experimental chemotherapeutic drug to dissolve the embryo. FGR president Twerdahl recognizes that with most medical treatments, patients are willing to take risks in order to gain benefits, but that in this case the donors receive no medical benefit. In addition, they will be taking drugs and may suffer side effects from them. The women who agree to be donors seem unconcerned about the risks and focus on the benefits that may result for infertile people. As one donor told us, "I'm proud to be part of this. I'd be proud to say, 'I helped her have a baby.'"

Twerdahl estimates that the average cost per OT cycle will be under $3,000, making it less expensive than hiring a surrogate or trying IVF. This amount represents an average of the high cost for screening the donor, the infertile woman, and her husband prior to the first cycle and the lower costs for subsequent cycles. Still, the cost will be prohibitive for most families, although insurance policies may cover some of the procedures.

Success Rate

How successful is the procedure? Dr. John Buster told us of a 60 percent success rate, but his published reports of the first trials are considerably more cautious. It is true that 60 percent of the blastocysts (the most developed fertilized ova) that were transferred resulted in pregnancies. However, only five blastocysts were recovered after eighteen months and fifty-three inseminations of ten donor women. Three pregnancies resulted (hence the 60 percent, or three out of five) but one ended in a miscarriage. It is striking that four of the five blastocysts came from only one donor, although all ten donor women had been carefully screened for fertility. This result demonstrates the high mortality of fertilized eggs. Twenty less-developed embryos were also transferred, but only one produced a pregnancy. This was an ectopic pregnancy, and the woman's tube had to be removed.[5]

During the first eighteen months that OT was attempted by Buster and his colleagues, thirteen women received embryos. Thirteen women, two babies. This may sound pretty good for a first trial. However, the donor and recipient women also experienced two miscarriages and an ectopic pregnancy. In addition, recipient women who had babies became pregnant within the first six months of the program. For another year until the research ended, and in subsequent trials at the Harbor campus, there has not been a single successful pregnancy.[6] This is hardly an outstanding success story. Yet the developers of the method point out that the initial trials were only the experimental phase.

With more donors, more drugs to eliminate retained pregnancies in the donors, and more money, they hope to limit the losses and improve the rates considerably.

On the basis of this very limited experience with thirteen women, Buster proclaimed that "the research is completed, the success of the procedure is proven," and plans for a national marketing campaign were launched. Good medical research, however, would seem to require a much larger sample, trials by other researchers, and better evidence of safety and effectiveness before making a procedure available to the general public. The American Fertility Society's ethics committee concluded in 1986 that, because of reservations about the procedure, OT should still be carried out only under carefully controlled experimental conditions.[7]

Commercialization of Fertility Treatment

"We're a technology company, just like any other. . . . We're no different from Polaroid or any other company that invents a new process and wants a patent to protect it."[8]

Lawrence Sucsy is an investment banker who has done much of the fund-raising for FGR. For him and many others in the financial field, infertility is a growth business, a booming market aimed at highly motivated and affluent consumers.

When the OT procedure was first publicized, and FGR made known its intention to seek patents for the catheter and the process, there was a great deal of criticism. Jeremy Rifkin, a leading opponent of genetic engineering, threatened to bring a lawsuit to contest the patent, claiming it "reduces the process of human reproduction to a consumer product to be bought and sold in the marketplace."[9] The medical community was equally opposed to FGR's approach to research. An attorney for the American Medical Association explained: "It's always been the view of the medical profession that you should have as widespread dissemination as possible of anything that would be beneficial to patients."[10]

Only a few years later, the criticism seems to have diminished somewhat. The American Fertility Society opposes the patenting of infertility procedures but not of the instruments themselves. And FGR is not the only infertility company trading on the stock market and setting up joint ventures for profit. Private infertility clinics offering a wide range of treatments are following the same path. Franchise operations are also appearing in the infertility field. As FGR president Twerdahl told us, referring to the growing willingness of medical institutions to consider joining the OT program: "At first they laughed at John Buster and then they ridiculed him. Now they think what we are doing is pretty serious medicine."

What difference does the form of organization make for infertile people? From the point of view of FGR's John Buster and James Twerdahl, exclusive control by a profit-making company can only make things better. They believe that this approach will guarantee high quality, a large enough pool of donors, and uniformity of performance from one place to another. According to Buster:

> The financial issues and the patient care issues and the quality issues are usually about the same. The company does well by contracting only with first class organizations. It will do well only if it serves the people well, if it is perceived as taking good care of the women. If not, it will fail.

Of course many corporations have done extremely well financially by treating their customers, workers, and neighbors very badly. If ovum transfer has any success, FGR will not *have* to treat people well, because infertile people will come to it anyway.

Buster also told us that, without private financing, the research for OT would never have been possible. He describes himself as having been driven into the arms of Wall Street types by the unavailability of funding:

> The alternative is to do nothing at all. Wall Street will never help you unless they get their money out. It's kind of analogous to going swimming with sharks. I mean, the sharks are pretty vicious, but their behavior is predictable and if you do exactly what they want and understand that predictable behavior, it is fine. You have to understand that getting money out of it is what makes their system work for them, even though that relationship compromises some of the dear academic principles we've always espoused.

Centralized control may in fact be an advantage, especially when compared to the very uneven performance of different IVF centers that have been started independently. Profit-making health programs, however, are not necessarily any more efficient or cost-effective than nonprofit ones. The incentives for them to cut corners and to concentrate on the most profitable activities are very strong. As Buster himself admits:

> There is a very delicate balance between keeping the Wall Street crew happy, keeping the physicians happy, and keeping the patients happy.

Ovum Transfer for Prenatal Diagnosis

For a few years, at least, ovum transfer will be used only to help infertile couples. In the future, however, if it achieves a high success rate, some of its developers foresee using the procedure for all pregnant women as a means of prenatal diagnosis.

Dr. Buster, the key researcher on the ovum transfer team, has moved on to new frontiers. His concern now is not with making babies but with improving their "quality." He described the embryo to us as a "little microchip," a package containing an incredible amount of information. Now he is researching that package, decoding the information to discover defects in the chip. According to Buster:

> In another five years infertility will be a nonissue, when there's an abundance of human ova available. Women are going to be much more concerned about the quality of life than they are about whether or not they can have babies.

Ovum transfer offers the technology to all women to diagnose their embryos before they even implant in the uterus. Women who are now advised to have prenatal testing must wait eight weeks for a chorionic villus sampling or sixteen weeks for amniocentesis and then agonize over the possibility of an abortion. With OT, they could have the newly fertilized egg checked after five days and reinserted in the uterus only if it is healthy.

Scientists such as John Buster claim that soon they will be able to detect not only genetic diseases in new embryos but even tendencies to diabetes, heart disease, and other disorders. Will all of the embryos with these problems be discarded? Will future children with the wrong color hair or shape of nose be tossed out, with the woman trying again the next month for a more perfect "package"? According to the scientists, no embryos will be discarded; instead, the defects will be repaired. We wonder, though, how many people would go to the expense and trouble of genetic repair of an embryo if it is relatively easy to produce a new one.

All of the reproductive technologies have this potential for applying eugenics to human procreation. They all will eventually allow parents to pick their children's characteristics. According to journalist Martin Stuart-Harle, Richard Seed, one of FGR's founders, believes that "there has always been a shortage of humans in Western civilization" and that OT could be a key to "the success of Western civilization."[11]

OT is not likely to contribute very much toward achieving this vision. It is more likely to be used by fertile women who are worried they might have handicapped children and who are able to monitor the possibility of a pregnancy from the very beginning. These would tend to be more affluent and educated women with access to the most advanced medical resources. They are the people who, if they have handicapped children now, push hard for better services. When only poor and uneducated women have children with serious problems, how much influence will they have over the allocation of resources to help such children?

♦ ♦ ♦ ♦ ♦

At the time of this writing, the commercial phase of ovum transfer is just beginning. The catheter has received a patent; the patent on the procedure is still pending. The experience to date raises many questions, but the answers may be known only in a few years. This relatively simple method, if it works, could prove to be a tremendous advantage for infertile women, allowing them to become pregnant with a minimum of risk and physical stress. The experience for donors, both physically and emotionally, is likely to be much more mixed. The implications for the future for all women who want children may be a great deal more far reaching.

Significant
Others

7
Donors and
Surrogate Mothers

Bob had not yet finished unpacking his bags when, glancing at the clock, he realized his first class was about to begin. As he sprinted across the quad, he felt the tension rising inside of him. It was the start of his second year of medical school, and everyone agreed that this year was the worst. Besides, the tuition had just gone up again. He felt he was being slowly sucked into a quicksand of debts. It was hard to imagine how he could make it through the next year.

As he passed the mailboxes, he noticed an official-looking letter inside and prayed that it would not be another bill. Instead, it was a letter from one of his professors in obstetrics and gynecology, telling him and the other men in his class about the need for sperm donors. The professor described the growing problem of male infertility, and, like a military recruiter, he ended with, "I'm looking for a few good men."

Bob stopped in his tracks, realizing that this might be a solution. He recalled later:

> The line that caught my eye was the one that said, "I will pay you $35 for every specimen." I thought, this could make a dent in my bills if I do it regularly! I looked at it as a lot easier than selling blood, which I was chicken to do anyway. Here was a way I could help people and do myself a favor at the same time. And frankly, I think I've got pretty good genes—I figured I'd be a great candidate.
>
> The letter said that if you're interested, fill out this form describing yourself—stuff like hair and eye color, height,

race, special interests. Then there was a medical history form—what did your grandmother die from, things like that. I had never been tested for genetic diseases like Tay-Sachs but I couldn't think of anyone in my family who's had a problem so I just said no to the question about genetic problems. Later I took a genetics course and realized that I had had no idea which diseases could be inherited or how.

It turned out to be so easy. As far I was concerned, the most difficult part was getting to the office early in the morning and getting out of there before the women arrived. I have to admit that I wondered about these women and their husbands. Occasionally I'd imagine this beautiful girl carrying my handsome baby. Most of the time, though, I just wanted to do my job, get my money, and be out of there to get to class on time.

I was glad when it ended after a year. I was starting to feel uncomfortable about possibly having so many children that I don't know. The closer I came to starting my own family, the more real the idea of fathering became for me.

Who Becomes a Donor or Surrogate Mother?

Who are the men and women we call donors? Who are these people who sell sperm, eggs or embryos, or who become pregnant for nine months in order to create a child for someone else? Why do they do it, and how do they feel about having children they may never know? The answers to these questions are different for male and female donors, and from one method to another.

Unfortunately, little is known about the donors. This is understandable in the case of egg and embryo donors because there are so few of them. There have been hundreds of surrogate mothers, however, over the last decade, and several studies of them exist.[1] There is a great deal of curiosity about who these women are and why they would become surrogates.

In contrast, there has been a lack of interest in sperm donors and their reasons for doing it, despite the fact that AID has been practiced for over one hundred years. Tens—if not hundreds— of thousands of men have sold their sperm in the United States alone during that time. Yet not a single American study of these men exists.

The lack of research on male donors says a great deal about the obsession with secrecy that surrounds AID. Most of what we do know about the feelings and motivations of sperm donors comes from anecdotal information, from interviews and informal contacts, and from a few studies carried out in other countries.[2]

We do know that, until recently, the vast majority of donors of fresh sperm in the United States were medical students or residents. In a 1979 survey of American physicians who perform AID, 85 percent reported using fresh sperm. Of these, more than three-fifths relied solely on medical students or residents, 10 percent on other students, and 18 percent on a combination of both.[3]

This picture is changing rapidly, however, as the demand for AID increases and sperm banks make frozen semen more available and easier for physicians to use. With frozen sperm, doctors no longer have to worry about screening the donors themselves or about the logistics of arranging for donors to be in the right place at the right time. With this development has come some change in the pool of donors. They are still selected for academic achievement, but not only in the medical field. They are also more likely to consider selling their semen as a long-term job.

Even with the changes in the field, the motives of sperm donors appear to have changed very little. Some are curious about their fertility, wondering if their sperm is any good. Others are motivated by sympathy for people who want children. For most men, however, the major reason to be a donor is the financial incentive.

Surveys in other countries such as Australia found many donors stating their willingness to continue even without payment. Yet where payments are low or nonexistent, as in France, it has been difficult to recruit men. One Australian physician who doubled the fee experienced an immediate increase in applicants.[4]

Money was the major factor for a law student named Ken, who saw an ad placed by a sperm bank. He thought this would be an easy way to buy the car he had always wanted. He said:

> I felt a little strange answering the ad. I told a few close friends I was thinking of doing this as a joke. We all laughed. When I went into the clinic they gave me a physical exam and had me masturbate in the bathroom to

examine my sperm. I then asked the doctor, "How does it look?" I always wondered how good my sperm really is. After looking at it under his microscope, he said, "So far it looks good, but we won't know until other tests, including a Karyotype for genetic information, are done."

A few weeks later they called and asked if I wanted to try being a donor. By then it wasn't a joke any more. I had decided to go ahead.

Ken has been a donor now for two years, and he figures he is making as much money for five minutes in the bathroom as he does for almost a whole day at his job as a law clerk. He takes his sperm donor job very seriously. He keeps himself in good shape, watching his weight and never smoking. He also makes sure not to have sex for forty-eight hours before giving his sperm.

Ken was proud of being one of the sperm bank's star donors. He recalled:

Until I started being a donor, I wasn't absolutely sure if I could get a woman pregnant. It turns out I must have been a super stud, because they asked me to do it a lot of times.

I wonder once in a while how many children I have out there in the world. Of course, I've never asked at the sperm bank—they probably don't even know and if they did, they wouldn't tell me anyway. Sometimes I try to calculate: if one child is produced every time I make a donation—let's see that would be about 112 children! Of course, that's unlikely.

What I do know for sure is that so far I've made $5,600, $50 every time. Not a bad record. The children don't feel real to me—it's as if they're not really there. But my car is, and every time I make another payment I feel great that the extra money helps me afford it.

If being a sperm donor is so easy and lucrative, why don't more men offer their services? According to one physician who recruits donors in a medical school, fifty letters from him can produce twenty responses one year but only three or four the next. The reluctance on the part of the majority must be more than a concern with inconvenience.

Some men may be put off primarily by their uneasiness about masturbation, especially on demand and in a hospital bathroom. Others fear that a child they never knew existed might come back one day to demand money or disrupt their lives. Many men are reluctant to father anonymous children, feeling some responsibility to care for, or at least to acknowledge, their offspring. The sociobiologists who claim that men are genetically programmed to maximize the number of children they create have never tried to recruit sperm donors.

Men who decide to become sperm donors may be kidded by their friends, but they do not have to face any serious social stigma. Also, it is possible to keep this activity secret from others if they want to. In Robyn Rowland's study of Australian sperm donors, 77 percent had told someone about being a donor. Yet 31 percent of those who were living with a partner had not told her and had no intention of telling her.[5]

For a man to sell his sperm and "father" unknown numbers of children for profit does not seem to disturb or intrigue the general public. When it comes to surrogate mothers, the situation is very different. The idea that a woman could give birth to a child for $10,000 and then give it away is considered "unnatural." Of course, giving up a baby after nine months of pregnancy *is* very different from a quick ejaculation of semen. The motivations of surrogate mothers are therefore very different from those of sperm donors.

Jenny is in many ways typical of women who decide to have a baby for someone else. She is married, with children, and had never heard about this type of program until one day she noticed an ad in the newspaper saying, "Surrogate mothers wanted to bear children for infertile couples." She recalls:

> I showed it to my husband just to see his reaction. I was surprised that he didn't oppose it. All he said was, "As long as you don't have to sleep with the guy, if you want to do it, it's OK."
>
> In the beginning I wanted to do it for the finances, because we were very much in debt. After carrying the baby, the money didn't matter so much. It was just the feeling of giving someone the gift of life. Maybe I was destined to see that ad and this is my part to give to humanity.

Women who become surrogate mothers emphasize their empathy for the infertile and their desire to do something special. Many of them love being pregnant but do not want any more children to take care of. For many, it is a chance to do something that fits with a traditional role—having a baby—but in a unique way. The first "generation" of surrogates has received a great deal of media attention, and for some women this is a big advantage. According to Nancy Reame at the University of Michigan, most surrogates are women who see few possibilities for satisfaction in their lives. "This is their one chance to shine."[6]

Surrogates are also a more varied group than sperm donors seem to be. According to Burton Satzberg, attorney for Surrogate Mothering Limited, in Philadelphia:

> The women, interestingly enough, have very little in common with each other. Some of them are highly educated, others are not; some fairly well off, and others are not. Different religions, different interests. Some are homebodies and some are out there in careers. The only things they have in common are that they enjoy being pregnant and they all have had very positive birth experiences.

Despite this variety of backgrounds, some patterns do emerge, partly due to program requirements. The majority are married, have one or two children, and have completed at least a high school education. They are strong minded and willing to do something that might be disapproved of. They are almost all white and Protestant or Catholic. Hilary Hanafin of Los Angeles describes the women she selects as "really neat people," who are emotionally healthy.

It is increasingly possible, with embryo or egg donation, for a woman to be a donor without carrying a baby to term. The donors for the OT program share some of the characteristics of surrogates. They are empathetic, often having a friend or relative who is infertile. The women who offered to be embryo donors for the first experimental round of OT are described by Annette Brodsky, a psychologist who screened them, as "not the average lady off the street." She found them to be adventurous, but also concluded that many were trying to make up for an unstable past. One OT donor explained to us why she likes what she is doing:

> It's a gift of God to pass on. It also helps me with self-confidence. I've always been shy and let other people walk all over me. When I was in school I had a lot of friends; then I got married and devoted myself to my husband, that was it. It makes me feel good to do something for somebody—every time I leave there I'm on a high. And where would we be today without guinea pigs?

Egg donors are least likely to be paid, but they are also not volunteers responding to an ad or a letter. Since the removal of eggs requires surgery, physicians ordinarily approach women who are already having surgery and ask them to donate some of their eggs. Women who are having hysterectomies or who are undergoing laparoscopies as part of IVF or other infertility treatments are the most likely candidates. According to physicians, such women are highly sympathetic to the problems of infertility and rarely say no. They certainly are in a vulnerable situation and would be reluctant to refuse their doctors' requests.

Now that donor programs are becoming less experimental and more routine, the characteristics of the donors are already changing. Those who are attracted by the potential for media attention and the desire to be pioneers may be less likely to apply. More donors will also be recruited by friends who have already been surrogates or donors rather than by newspaper and television ads. Some surrogate programs are reporting that more highly educated and emotionally stable women are now applying than in the past.

The Ideal Donor, the Ideal Surrogate

We asked program staff and couples to describe what they were looking for in an ideal donor. Although health was always a major factor, the other priorities differed greatly depending on whether they needed a male or a female donor. The differences were closely tied to sex role stereotypes.

Most programs that need sperm donors, for example, look for intelligent men. The profiles of donors at IDANT Laboratories, a New York sperm bank that is the largest in the United States, include grade point averages, and 3.5 to 4.0 is common. An extreme example of this requirement for intelligence is seen in the policies of the Repository for Germinal Choice in Escondido, California (better known as the Nobel sperm bank). It dedicates itself to improving the human race by using only donors who have superior intelligence.

In contrast, when it comes to surrogate mothers, qualities such as stability, warmth, openness, physical attractiveness, strength of character, and compassion are considered more important than intelligence. All surrogate programs screen applicants for psychological makeup. We are aware of only one program, in Belgium, that screens potential sperm donors psychologically and turns away those considered to be unstable.[7] The difference is striking. The father should be intelligent, the mother should be nurturing and pretty.

Some of these criteria are logical. Surrogate mothers certainly give a great deal more of themselves to the baby, and often to the couple as well, than do sperm donors, and that does make personality traits, at least, much more important. However, the case of women donors in the OT program supports the view that powerful stereotypes are at play as well. The role of the women donors in that program is in many ways similar to the role of sperm donors. They are often anonymous, and their involvement is much more short term. Yet they are screened like surrogates, with a great deal of attention to personality and psychological stability. Intelligence is not an important factor.

The difference in priorities when selecting a male versus a female donor is based on a traditional view of the ideal father and the ideal mother. Perhaps the professionals who do the screening and the prospective parents as well are trying to create a balance they assume a child born of the two of them would have. Perhaps at some level they also assume that a surrogate mother will give birth to a girl, who should be very "feminine" and that AID will lead to a son, who had better be "masculine."

Findings One's Own Donor

More people are deciding to do without the professional "matchmakers" who recruit and screen donors and manage the relationship among all the parties. They prefer to select their own egg donor, sperm donor, or surrogate, in the last two cases often performing the insemination themselves. One survey found that 63 percent of the medical students studied and 78 percent of a sample of infertility support group members agreed that AID recipients should be allowed to select their own donors.[8] This statistic is surprising in light of the current prevailing practice of anonymity.

There are some advantages to finding one's own donor. It avoids the control and the biases of professionals and is almost always less expensive. Noel Keane, the lawyer who started the first surrogate mother program, was introduced to the idea by a couple who were having a young unmarried friend carry a baby for them and needed an attorney to handle the legal aspects. He still helps couples who recruit their own surrogate, charging them less than his usual fee.

Another reason many prefer to choose their own donors, especially with AID, is so their children will have the option of knowing who their father is and having contact with him if they want. Some known sperm donors do in fact take a part in the child's life.

Having a donor who knows the mother is not always an advantage. He may want more involvement with the child than the mother (or her husband). Occasionally the mother and the donor end up in court battling over visitation and custody. Single women, heterosexual as well as lesbian, are particularly vulnerable because courts have ruled in the man's favor when there was not another man around to be the father.[9]

The problems become even more complicated when family members are involved. As one woman said:

My sister offered to have a baby for me. She figured it would be ideal, because the baby would have genes like mine and she would still be Aunt Betty just as if I had given birth to the child. But as great an idea as it is in theory, I knew it would be a disaster. She's the kind of person who would want to be telling me how to raise the kid, and never let me forget what she did. I'd rather have someone who isn't so close to me.

Sometimes having a relative be a surrogate mother or sperm donor does work well. Even before the national media publicized the case of a woman who bore a child for her sister, family members were already making such private arrangements. A close relative, a brother or sister, is likely to offer empathy as well as genetic similarity. There may be disputes over parenting or conflicts with the donor's spouse, but we have heard of several instances of women having babies for sisters and still maintaining close relationships between the two families.

Lesbian couples often find their own donor in order to avoid the scrutiny of professionals. One gay woman who tried to find her own donor discovered that it was more difficult than she expected. She said:

We got turned down, I don't know how many times. They'd say, "Oh, I don't know if I could handle it." "Nobody's asking you to handle anything," we said, "just give us your sperm!" We weren't asking for any financial support, the kid didn't even have to ever know who they were. We had a lawyer ready to sign every legal document in the whole world. We were all prepared. But they'd say, "But I'd just know that there was this child." We were so angry that they couldn't just give us sperm—two seconds you know.

Occasionally a woman who wants to be a surrogate mother looks for a couple herself. One woman placed an advertisement in the newspaper offering to have a baby for an infertile couple.

Since private arrangements with donors are unrecorded and therefore unstudied, we cannot know how frequently this happens or how well it works. Certainly as artificial insemination, ovum transfer, and surrogate motherhood become more widespread, more public, and therefore more acceptable, these informal arrangements will become increasingly common.

The matchmakers who run programs prefer, of course, that the selection be left up to them. One surrogate program director, for example, reasoned that the careful safeguards involved in his screening procedure are essential. Certainly, a thorough health screening is important, but there is no reason that an individual or couple could not arrange to have a donor screened. It is also true that the screening of donors by physicians is not always as rigorous as it should be.

Risks for Embryo Donors and Surrogates

People who become donors usually talk about the positive side of their experience. They feel good about helping others, and the extra money can be a big help. There are risks as well, however. The risks are particularly great for the women donors, both embryo donors and surrogates. They face a multitude of physical risks, ranging from the minor discomforts of pregnancy to possible (though rare) death from ectopic pregnancy or childbirth. They are artificially inseminated with sperm that may not be carefully screened, exposing themselves to the possibility of infections, venereal disease, or even AIDS, which threaten health, future fertility, or life itself.

Annette Brodsky explains why embryo donors might ignore these risks:

> Some donors say: "I trust this program, I trust the people, if they think it's OK, and they've researched it, and they've looked at it, then I'll be OK." We tell them all the risks—we can't let them out of here without knowing. But, there's a lot of not wanting to know.

One risk of concern to some women who become surrogates is the possibility the couple may reject a child if he or she is born with a handicap. In one highly publicized case in this country, the baby was born with microcephaly, indicating a likelihood of retardation. The presumed father questioned whether the baby was his and raised the possibility that he would not take the child. The results of blood tests announced in front of a national audience on the "Donahue" show revealed that the surrogate's husband was actually the father, and she agreed to keep the baby. However, if the surrogate's husband had not been the biological father, the question of who would raise the baby would probably not have been decided as easily.

A much more common problem for surrogate mothers is the emotional trauma of giving up the baby. One woman described her own experience:

> Through the whole pregnancy I was motivating myself, trying to put my state of mind into what I wanted it to be for the delivery and after. But it was still very hard, that separation, much harder than I thought it would be. I wonder how she's doing, what kind of life she'll have. I wish I had thought to ask the couple if I could be the guardian of the baby if anything happened to them. But I know I have to try not to think about her. Her birthday is especially hard. I always get depressed then.
>
> I wanted to keep in touch with the baby's parents—after all, we had gotten to know each other pretty well and you'd think they'd want to know how I am. We had agreed from the beginning that after the baby was born we would not contact each other. But I hadn't realized how hard it would be saying good-bye to them. I haven't heard from them since that day we said good-bye.

Surrogates face grief from loss of the baby and frequently from the loss of their connection with the couple. Psychiatrist Philip

Parker, in his follow-up study of thirty surrogate mothers, found several who had severe grief reactions and required treatment.[10] One of the first surrogate mothers, "Elizabeth Kane," who publicly stated how easy it was to give up her baby, appeared on television seven years later to express her remorse. She now feels that she and her other children have been damaged by the surrogate arrangement.

As surrogate programs are increasingly combined with IVF, the emotional dimension for surrogate mothers may change somewhat. In these cases a woman becomes pregnant with the embryo of a couple, and she may feel more like a "hired womb." A woman who was trying to conceive with frozen embryos explained her feelings about it:

> This has nothing to do with me at all. It's not my egg and it's not my husband's sperm. I'll be an incubator, that's really what it is. You know I'm just going to take care of their baby, like babysitting it for nine months. It's kind of long to babysit somebody, but that's the way I look at it.

What will it mean for women to carry and give birth to babies who are not "theirs" genetically, yet who have been part of their bodies for nine months? Will it really be easier, or is that another form of self-deception to suit the needs of others? After nine months of the most intimate connection, we'd be surprised if it weren't just as hard to give up a baby, regardless of its genes.

The emotional risks for surrogate mothers may be eased by professional counseling, but it is rarely after the baby is relinquished. Some surrogates feel that seeing the happy family together helps them cope with the loss. But what about those women who never see the baby again and do not know where he or she is? They do their best to detach themselves from the experience and go on with their lives. Do they repress grief, only to see it emerge again months or years later? No one knows the answers yet.

There may be risks for the surrogate's family life as well, something about which we do not yet have reliable information. For instance, many surrogates said their husbands were very supportive. Is it really irrelevant to these husbands that their wives are pregnant from the sperm of other men, especially affluent, well-educated men who the surrogates have come to believe will make great fathers? Will the marriage suffer if the woman feels her husband pushed her into being a surrogate for the money? Can their other children really understand that "Mommy is babysitting Ray and Betsy's baby for nine months because Betsy's tummy doesn't work" and not wonder how Mommy could give away their baby sister or brother? What will be the long-term effects on these children?

The women we interviewed felt confident that, so far, their families had not suffered. They gave instances instead of how encouraging their husbands and other relatives had been, how easily the other children had accepted the situation. Until follow-up studies are done, there will be no way to know how many women, or members of their families, suffer long-term damaging effects.

Some women donors mention as a benefit the attention they receive from prestigious people. They are courted and cared for—if only temporarily—by physicians and lawyers, and may even appear on television. This need for attention may ultimately backfire. Program staff remark that some women return regularly for favors and advice, expecting to receive continued support. They do not always get what they are looking for and end up feeling angry and disappointed.

One woman, whose experience as a surrogate mother can only be described as destructive, is ready to do it again because of her continuing need for approval by the program directors:

> The pregnancy made me feel sick as a dog, I've never been so sick in my life. I was going through a great deal of emotional problems and admitted myself to a hospital to get some rest. I had to place my children in foster homes for the rest of the pregnancy.
>
> The pregnancy kept me going through all that, and also my relationship with the program. I would trust those guys with my life. They really care about me, they tell me I'm their star. They're my knights in shining armor; they've helped me through a lot. Even though I'm having a hard time getting pregnant again, I'll keep trying for them.

Hilary Hanafin, who counsels women for a Los Angeles surrogate program, suggests that some women may actually benefit from being surrogates. She said:

> It's not unusual to hear that a surrogate has decided to go back to school and finish her degree, or put a down pay-

ment on a house she's always wanted. I think it's a combination of finances and of also having achieved something unique that really gives them that boost, that transition from being a housewife to attacking another career.

Risks for Sperm Donors

Physicians who work with artificial insemination or who have donated sperm themselves do not believe there are any emotional problems associated with donating sperm. If there is any risk, it is that a child may find the donor father who would prefer to remain anonymous. There have in fact been a number of children who have tried to trace their fathers through medical school records or yearbooks.

The chance of this happening, however, is still small. Most of the children do not know of their AID origins, and if they do, the possibility of finding the biological father is slim. Records are poorly kept or destroyed. Only in Sweden is it required that a record be kept of the donor and that children have the right to this information after they reach the age of eighteen.

A surprising number of donors would like to have contact with the children, or at least would not mind it. Robyn Rowland, in her study of Australian sperm donors, discovered that 60 percent of her sample would not mind meeting the children they had fathered. Forty-two percent claimed that they would still donate even if their names were given to the couple.[11]

Often it is the donor's wife who is more concerned. She may worry that some of her husband's dozens of offspring may come looking for him, perhaps threatening her own children's well-being as well as their inheritance.

Donors and Recipients

The great majority of donors and recipients have no contact and very little knowledge about each other because secrecy until now has been the rule for AID and OT. Surrogate programs vary widely in their policies, from those that forbid any contact between surrogate and couple to others that require it. Of course in the case of IVF, where usually no donor is involved, there is no problem with secrecy. Yet when donors, whether of eggs or sperm, are brought into IVF, they are almost always anonymous.

Professionals who advocate secrecy sometimes justify it by claiming that a relationship between donor and recipients would intensify fantasies about each other, which could lead to trouble. According to psychologist Howard Adelman of Surrogate Mothering Limited:

> If the surrogate meets the couple there's the possibility of fantasies starting. She starts really liking this guy who is the father, and maybe thinking she'd like to have this child of his and keep it and even—in very unrealistic situations—possibly he'll leave his wife for her. So when they ask what he looks like, I make a joke out of it—I say, "He's very short, fat with a big belly, and bald," and they laugh.

Anonymity, however, offers no guarantee of eliminating troublesome fantasies. Perhaps it is harder to act on them, but they may actually be exaggerated by lack of reality. Donors and recipient couples who never meet often have fears and fantasies about each other. Many times these revolve around racial or religious prejudices. Fantasies about other characteristics are often present as well. "I hope he doesn't look like John Belushi," a woman commented after being inseminated.

Some people who advocate secrecy in a surrogate program fear that the birth mother will "blackmail" the couple later in order to receive more money. In addition, anonymity has the advantage of diminishing the couple's sense of obligation to do more for someone who has given them such an important gift.

The major argument against secrecy is the same one used in discussions of adoption—harm to the children who may want or need to know their parentage. In addition, many surrogates want to know the families to whom they are giving their babies. Like other birth mothers who give up babies for adoption, they need to know where the babies are and how they are doing.

One woman surrogate who developed a close relationship with the adoptive couple described the reasons for her feelings about contact with the child:

> I was adopted and knew my birth mother, and I realized that I couldn't handle anonymity. So we decided before I even got pregnant that it was very important that the child know who I am and feel comfortable enough to call me if

he felt the need to talk to me, that he would have that right to do it.

This woman has already visited the child twice and speaks to the parents regularly by phone. Their situation, however, is not very common.

One element present in most relationships is the payment. Whether it be $30 for a sperm donor or $10,000 for a surrogate, very few people become involved with one of these methods for free. As George Annas, professor at Boston University Law School, points out, it would be more accurate to call them vendors instead of donors.[12]

There are pluses and minuses with payment, just as with secrecy. Both appear to increase the likelihood that a sufficient number of donors will be available. Both present difficult conflicts for many of the people involved.

In his classic study of blood donation, *The Gift Relationship,* Richard Titmuss found that those countries in which blood donors are paid have major problems with donors concealing information that would have disqualified them.[13] The same may be true for sperm donors, who have been known to split one sample of semen into more than one donation, and also to misrepresent their medical histories.

Some people who do not really want to be donors may feel compelled to do so because of their need for money. Payment is also troubling because of the implications of "baby selling." In an ideal world, people would give of themselves for altruistic reasons, to help others in need. Unfortunately, we have seen from the experience of other countries such as France, where donors are not paid, that altruism is rarely enough of an incentive to begin to meet the demand for donors.

◆　◆　◆　◆　◆

Often donors enter into a program as a lark, or from financial need. And often they discover that they are giving a very precious gift, one that may make others incredibly happy. Many couples told us about their feelings of gratitude, feelings they usually never get a chance to express to the donors:

> I love my son with all my heart. But I can't forget that a stranger played an essential role in my child's conception.

Without him, my son would not exist. I know we'll never meet the donor, but sometimes I wish he could visit us and see for himself what a precious human being he has helped to create.

8
The Professionals

It had been a particularly rough day for Dr. B., the director of a fertility center. He shut the door of his office, sat back in his big leather chair, and sighed. He was clearly exhausted. He was willing to be interviewed about his work, but he was distracted by thoughts of the phone call he had just made. He explained:

A couple came in last year who had had two children; she then had a tubal ligation. Later one of the children died and she wanted to have another. Tubal surgery didn't work, so IVF was their only chance. She told me they were people of meager means. They had sold their second car and raised $10,000. They figured that, with insurance, they had enough for three chances. "Here we are, Doc," they said, looking at me with hope in their eyes. Today I got the third negative pregnancy test. I just feel the lowest of low. It's really, really tough.

If I think too much about every patient's pain and sacrifices, I wouldn't be able to focus on developing new procedures that may help them. If I spend more time consoling and talking to them, there will be no time for the next person. I know they're angry and desperate, but I just can't always deal with it.

The hardest part of my work is trying to treat such a large number of patients. It requires such extraordinary patient-physician interaction, so much emotional energy involved in it, and after a while, it is wearing. My God, they are all lined up out there—one side of my brain says I'm obliged to treat every person that I can and the other side says, if you treat any more, you won't even know their names.

People who try the new methods have entrusted their futures to powerful individuals. They bring to these physicians and lawyers their hopes and anxieties, their vulnerable overtested bodies, and often their life savings. They seek understanding and compassion, information and support, and most of all, of course, they seek a baby. What they find is that the professionals they depend on often fail to understand their emotional needs. These professionals frequently focus only on the technical or legal details and do not realize how crucial their support is.

The Professionals and Their Motives

Who are these people who are offering the reproductive alternatives? Two entirely different images emerge from what has been written about them. In one image, commonly found in the media, these are extremely hardworking, imaginative, and dedicated people. They are creative scientists, empathetic attorneys, and caring physicians and nurses, devoting enormous energy to helping unfortunate couples achieve their most precious goal. They are pioneers, miracle workers, even saints.

There is also another image, painted by those who are critical of the new methods. They write of the "pharmacrats," the egomaniacal madmen whose search for fame and fortune is exploiting women today and may ruin society in the future. In this view, the infertility professionals are single-minded devotees of "science" who pursue "progress" without regard for the human and social consequences. Hiding behind the mask of benevolence, they are the manipulators and controllers of women.

Both pictures have some truth to them. In our interviews with professionals, we observed the complex merging of these two images. We met individuals who are motivated by the challenge of working at the frontiers of science and by the prestige of being at the top of their field. They are ambitious go-getters who feel there is no reason to be concerned about the present risks to women and possible future dangers. At the same time, they work very hard to help infertile couples. They share in the joys and disappointments of their clients and cannot understand why they would be considered exploiters of women.

When we asked directors of infertility and surrogate programs why they became involved in this kind of work, their answers usually centered on scientific and career concerns. The lure of scientific discovery, the chance to be a pioneer, is a principal motivation for many professionals. As one director of a fertility program put it:

> My thing in life is not to be just in the front running: I want to be right out there in the very front. The grant money in my area dried up; so I became interested in infertility. Personally, it is important to me that the work I do helps women. But by far the most exciting part professionally is the research and the new data we get.

Another physician remarked:

> Delivering babies became too routine for me—it just wasn't very creative. But IVF is really an exciting intellectual problem. It has unlimited potential.

Dr. Alan DeCherney, director of Reproductive Endocrinology at Yale University School of Medicine, represents this viewpoint most vividly. He wrote:

> We can only be overjoyed ... to be working during a period of time when such paramount advances have been made. How thrilling it must have been to be Chaucer writing when Gutenberg invented the printing press, or to be a physicist working on the Manhattan Project! ... An individual who is interested in fertility, who is not involved in IVF, is very similar to the West Point graduate who is educated in Military Science but never goes to war.[1]

There is something very troubling about the imagery here. The physician is compared to a warrior; the researchers on women's bodies are similar to the creators of the atomic bomb. The prestige and satisfaction of discovery, and the possibility of developing and using new skills, appear to be more important than helping women become pregnant.

The other side of this picture is that these same academically inclined professionals derive a tremendous satisfaction from the personal side of their work. For some, the desire to help people who are infertile had led them into this specialty in the first place. One infertility specialist explained:

> When I was a resident, my wife and I became friendly with the couple next door in our apartment building. She had a fertility problem and needed somebody to give her a Pergonal shot. That was how I learned about the terrible pain of infertility, and it was the dawn of my new career.

Another physician recalled:

> I was working with infertile couples, and it was so frustrating to always be saying, "There's nothing else to be done." I joined an IVF program so that I *could* offer more.

Does it make a difference why these professionals went into the field of infertility? After all, without driven scientists and entrepreneurial lawyers, there would be fewer options for the infertile. And from the point of view of people trying to have children, the motivations of providers may not appear to be important, as long as they can achieve success.

However, these physicians and lawyers are powerful people who hold the fate of many families in their hands and in their laboratories. If their priorities are science or prestige or financial gain, they should not be entrusted with decision making about the future of these procedures. And in the short run, it may be difficult for them to provide the needed emotional support for their clients.

The Power of Professionals

The professionals' power extends to many aspects of the methods. They decide who will be allowed into a program and what their experience will be like. They determine what procedures will be used and how much information the clients will have. They select the surrogate mothers or the donors and decide what new directions the research will take. The only control they do not have is over the outcome.

Control over access to services is an important source of power. There is no open-door policy with the new methods; every program sets criteria for screening clients. Marital status, age, fertility history, and emotional stability are usually considered before someone is allowed to try an alternative.[2] The ability to pay is the only standard shared by every program.

Many infertile people never get inside the well-guarded gates of fertility programs. The professional gatekeepers in many programs have declared them to be too old, too poor, too single, too far down on the waiting list, too neurotic, or medically unqualified. Some of the restrictions were instituted because the programs were new and the directors were worried about public relations. They believed that by accepting only married couples who were psychologically stable they would avoid bad publicity.

The psychological testing is the one aspect of the screening that bothers applicants the most. One woman recalled her session angrily:

> We had a horrible experience. The coordinator refused to tell me over the phone what the assessment was about and insisted that we just come in for the appointment. Additionally, we had to pay *in advance* and our check had to arrive before we went through the program. In retrospect, I should have been suspicious then. The actual assessment included intrusive, lengthy questionnaires about our sexual practices (questions beyond imagination!). A final interview with a psychologist revealed that this was a research study to determine if couples applying for IVF had sexual problems as well. She assured us that she didn't think that this was the case, and that as a group she found us "disgustingly normal." There seems to be an attitude among professionals that we are experimental guinea pigs even though we are paying (and the price is high) for the opportunity to try something with no guarantees or assurances.

Psychological screening may help patients to consider whether they can cope with the stress of the procedures. It may also, however, reinforce the emotional distress of the infertile couple who, already feeling inadequate, must prove their qualifications for parenthood. This is a challenge never presented to those who can conceive on their own; infertile people may wonder why they have to meet higher standards than other prospective parents.

According to the studies of couples who have applied to AID and IVF programs, very few have ever been rejected for psychological reasons. Some couples voluntarily change their minds after a full discussion of their motivations and plans; a few are referred for further counseling.[3] But the fact of screening gives a great deal of power to the physicians. Even though they do not turn away many couples, they could.

When there were not many programs available and few of them had a reputation for success, the long waiting lists became the greatest obstacle to acceptance. At one point a staff member of the Norfolk IVF program, for instance, estimated that it would take ten years to accommodate everyone already on the waiting list. In this kind of situation, assertiveness and personal connections often help move a name to the top of the list. Physicians may favor their own and their friends' patients, and lawyers may turn first to the couples they know or like the best.

Now that there is a great deal more competition for clients, and the public appears to be more accepting, the waiting lists are shorter and the standards for admission have become less rigorous. Age ceilings are slowly lifting, more programs are willing to accept single women, and psychological screening is less common.

Some physicians feel that their role in "gatekeeping" should be limited to giving the facts. One fertility specialist who practices AID told us:

> If a woman comes in here and she is unmarried, or a lesbian couple comes in and they decide they are in a stable relationship and want a child, who am I to decide that they shouldn't? My job is to inform them of the dangers and ask if they've thought about all the possibilities. If they have, I'm just playing a technician at that point. They could just as easily go to a bar and have sex with somebody to get pregnant. They might as well do it in a controlled manner.

Even the most liberal professionals, such as this doctor, see control as an essential part of their role.

Most people entering programs in which there is a donor trust the professionals to screen out problems effectively. For example, most women who tried AID told us they were sure that the sperm donors had been medically screened. Yet we have seen that selection is based more on academic accomplishment, and health is often checked very poorly. On the other hand, a women who had a baby as a surrogate mother told us she was certain the adoptive couple was screened for suitability as parents. Yet the director of the program that recruited her told us that if couples can afford it, they are accepted. He sends only surrogate applicants to the psychologist, never the couples.

Sociologist Marcia Millman describes the ways in which physicians "enact trust" from their patients. By withholding information and discouraging questions, they force patients and their families to fall back on the belief that the physician will do the right thing.[4] While some degree of confidence is important between patient and doctor, blind trust can be harmful. One woman said:

> I've had four laparoscopies in the last four years. I wouldn't think of changing doctors, even though I still haven't gotten pregnant. I think part of that is just the way I trust my doctor—if he wanted to cut me anywhere I'd say, "Fine, go ahead, do what you want."

Denial is a powerful force for self-protection in humans. It protects people from seeing or feeling what they would rather avoid. It is all the more powerful when reinforced by a lifetime of learning that one should trust people in authority, especially doctors. So when a kindly physician or psychologist tells someone that what he or she is about to do—whether it be open heart surgery or ovum donation—has possible risks, most people have learned not to listen. They trust that it will not happen to them.

Another concern about the control of professionals is related to the potential link between these methods and a growing movement called eugenics. People who believe in eugenics want to "improve" the population by limiting the reproduction of "inferior" people. Since it is the doctors and lawyers who choose prospective parents, donors, and surrogate mothers, will they decide to produce only babies with superior intellect or other specific characteristics? This is already happening, particularly in the way sperm donors are now selected for intellectual ability.

Perhaps the greatest power of these practitioners is the control they have over the creation of new life. "We are truly playing God," a psychologist with an IVF program told us.

Meeting the Needs of Clients

The professionals who work in fertility programs are crucial in the lives of the people who go to them for help. It is not surprising, then, that they evoke such strong emotions, both positive and negative. These conflicting comments from two women who had been through IVF are typical:

They were incredible human beings, always there for me. I think of them as family. They really helped me get through the hard times.

I didn't feel that they were very understanding about the pain I was in. We were dealt with as objects, as guinea pigs. Not that they wanted to; they just didn't have the staff. They didn't have the training. We were just numbers to them—it was much too impersonal.

Many professionals—attorneys, physicians, and staff—are very caring to their clients; just as often they are viewed as distant and lacking in understanding. Often they simply do not know how to deal with the emotions of people struggling with infertility. Unfortunately, their comments and attitudes have a tremendous impact. An unsympathetic staff person can intensify the stresses of an already difficult process. One woman was very upset about her doctor, who had said, "Why do you deserve to have a baby?" She explained that he had six children and thought that the better the person, the more children God would give you. A woman who was having artificial insemination was also very upset with her physician. She said:

It's hard for anyone to meet your emotional needs, but the one person who did the least of any one I know was my doctor. First of all, he had pregnant women in the waiting room at the same time I was there. And then he would hardly talk to me. When I complained one time, he said that he had thirty other women out there in his office just as anxious as I was and he had to see all of them in one hour. I really didn't have a choice because he was the only one in our area doing inseminations.

It would infuriate me when he would unexpectedly go out of town and not have anyone cover for him. Here I was planning my whole life around this schedule, I would be ovulating and he would be out of town. He said he couldn't ask another doctor to cover for him because then the donor would be known to someone else. I felt that if he was offering a service, he really owed it to the people to be there. However, he was more concerned about the donor than about his patients.

Lack of understanding, lack of time, lack of personalized attention. There are the themes that recur in the comments of people who have tried the alternative methods. We asked people what, if anything, they would change about the program they were in. By far the most frequent response was that it should provide more emotional support and counseling. There are so many pressures, expectations, frustrations, and feelings of isolation and anger, it is no wonder that a person would benefit from a professional counselor and from more contact with other couples. Though some receive the help they need from program staff, or from informal support groups, most people feel that more is required.

Formal support groups are rare for most programs because funds are scarce or because staff members believe there is no need for them. For example, Dr. Howard Jones of the Jones Institute of Reproductive Medicine in Norfolk claimed in a speech that IVF patients have no special emotional needs compared to other infertility patients and therefore programs to provide support are unnecessary.[5] In other programs, support groups have been announced, but they met at inconvenient times or were not presented as an essential part of the program. Under such circumstances, it is not surprising that they failed. At one university hospital, a more formal group has been set up where couples are encouraged to attend as part of the program. In addition, every couple is introduced to one or two other couples as a buddy system for support.

People going through these programs need support and contact from the staff at all stages of the process. They also need to be prepared for the possibility of failure. Feelings of isolation and depression are especially acute during waiting periods and after conception fails.

While the relationship between staff and patients may often be very good and helpful as long as the patients are physically at the program, this support often vanishes once they go home. One woman recalled her feelings:

> After the eight embryos were implanted and I went home, I felt the staff were very far away. I would call up and they would seem very, very distant—it seemed like they were billions of miles away. They were very curt and would say, "Send in your blood and we'll find out the results."

Many people told us they felt they were not getting from the professional staff honest information about the procedure and their realistic chances of success. They needed accurate information to make their decisions and were angry if they felt they had been misled. One man who wrote to us was furious when he learned, after his wife had gone through IVF, that her chances of success had been only 1 percent:

> After the fact we were told we were admitted because the clinic personnel thought that it was psychologically beneficial to experience failure, to which I say, "Hogwash!"

When their needs are met, even if the treatment is not successful, the gratitude is boundless. An example is a woman who gave birth after three attempts at IVF in the Norfolk clinic. She spoke about the founders, Drs. Georgeanna and Howard Jones:

> I'll never forget the fact that the Joneses were there. You know, she held my hand and patted my back during the transfer, and he did the transfer. I think of them as our child's grandparents.

One couple who were trying AIH told how appreciative they were of their doctor's dedication. The husband said:

> After three months of trying, we told him the procedure was too expensive for us to continue. We were surprised when he quickly said he would cut the fee in half. He's just doing everything he can to get us a baby—not everything he can to get a large bank account.

The physician who made extra visits in the hospital to a woman whose family was far away, the hospital staff who made a couple feel welcome in the delivery room while a surrogate mother gave birth to a child for them, the doctor who opened his office on Christmas to do an insemination, the receptionist who kept a woman company for the three hours she had to lie still after an embryo transfer, the nurse whose humor and friendliness made it possible to get through another day of tests and uncertainty—these people are remembered forever.

Stresses on Professionals

Infertility programs are certainly stressful for staff members as well as for the people who are infertile. The emotional difficulties for the professionals, however, are even less well recognized.[6]

Because the professionals have so much of their training and energy invested in these programs and so many people counting on them, they are often faced with difficult emotional stresses as well as technical challenges. They know that people are using up their retirement funds or the money they had saved for buying a house. They know they are frequently targets for the anger and frustration of the people they are trying to help. The pressure for success is intense.

For some, the frustrations arise mainly from the technical challenges. For example, several IVF physicians told us that the single most difficult aspect of their work was the situation where they did a laparoscopy and were not able to retrieve any eggs. It means that something went wrong in the process of monitoring hormone response. They feel more responsible at that point. It also seems more final than when a woman at least has some eggs that can be fertilized, even if she does not get pregnant on a given cycle.

Often the nurse coordinator of an IVF program is the one who is most intensely involved with couples. Joan is one such nurse; she has been part of a busy IVF center for two years. She described her role in the program:

> I get involved with every couple. It's hard not to, because the nurse is the person they see every single day. I'm the constant in the whole process. I'm the "good news, bad news" person. Everything goes through me. I see them every morning following their ultrasound and talk with them on the phone every evening with the results and instructions. I'm available at home if they need to call me for any reason.
>
> Yes, you do get wrapped up in it. It's very hard for me to call a patient with a negative pregnancy test. Emotionally it's the most difficult part of the job. But then there's the elation of calling those women who have a positive pregnancy test. I think I experience the same kind of emotional roller coaster they are experiencing because I want so much for it to be successful for every couple.

One of the toughest situations for people working in these programs is when their efforts are frustrated by a change of heart, such as the surrogate mother who decided to keep the baby, the woman who was so nauseous during her pregnancy following AID that she decided to have an abortion, or the IVF patient who went through hormone treatments only to refuse to undergo the laparoscopy because she had already experienced so much failure in her life and was afraid to fail again.

Professionals who work in surrogate or AID programs are less troubled than IVF or OT staff people by the difficulty of achieving a pregnancy. They are matching up two people who have no known fertility problems, and therefore they ordinarily see high rates of pregnancy. Their frustrations are more with the logistics of making the match—recruiting sperm donors and coordinating their schedules with the recipient women's cycles, or finding women who would be good surrogate mothers.

Programs that carefully screen surrogate mothers are caught in the difficult situation of needing women and yet sending many applicants away. The staff members feel stressed by the responsibility of making sure no one is hurt. Being in a situation for which there is little precedent also creates stress, as noted by Dorie McArthur, a psychologist who works with surrogates:

> The hardest part is that every week we consider an ethical, legal, philosophical, social issue for which there is no answer in any book. We're just ordinary human beings in this world, trying to figure out how to do it in a way that won't backfire. If it does backfire, what will the repercussions be? When do we take the risk and when do we not?

How do staff members deal with the stress? IVF programs, in particular, have informal supports for the team members. They take breaks between cycles, rely on the social worker or psychologist on the team to provide help, or they find contacts with other programs. One nurse coordinator found relief from the stress and pressures of her job by phoning a woman who had the same job at a different IVF clinic. She said:

> For a year, we were best friends on the phone. It was so great because we could really support each other. Her pregnancies really helped me when we had none. And when she was down, when she went through a real grief, a real dry spell, then my pregnancies helped her.

For some, the ability to keep going comes from the patients and their own inner strength. Another nurse said:

When I have to give bad news, they feel almost as bad for me as I do for them, so it's more of an "Oh, my God, what are we going to do?" feeling. They know I'm feeling bad. I also do a lot of blocking—that's my defense mechanism, and a lot of joking. Laughter is my way out instead of crying.

Do these professionals feel that they are special, that they are involved in creating life? For some, there is a thrill in making new life possible. They feel a special tie to the children, maintaining a long-term relationship like that of an aunt or uncle. A lawyer who runs a surrogate agency described the satisfaction he derives from his work:

There's such a fulfillment when you hand that baby over from the surrogate to the couple. It does feel like I'm part of creating life. You just look back and think these people had absolutely nothing till they came to us, and look what we've given them. It's something you just don't get in the practice of law. In practicing law you might get someone a bigger settlement, but in a few weeks it's going to be spent or put in the bank. That's nothing to compare with making a family.

Other professionals say they think about their work as being just like any other form of medicine. The director of an IVF program claimed that the procedure has received too much attention:

It is a normal treatment of infertility, and if you do it every day, it becomes a part of your daily work. We're not creating life, we're just making it possible for two germ cells to meet where otherwise they might not meet. It's just a normal extension of nature.

When we asked people who work with alternative methods what they like best about their work, the two dimensions—driven scientist and caring professional—appeared often. For some, it was the prestige of finding a new technique or the challenge of overcoming a difficult technical problem. For others, it was the excitement of a woman becoming pregnant. In the answer of one doctor:

What's the most satisfying part? Oh, my God, that's easy. Easy—the joy of those people.

Effects on
the Family

9
The Couple

*Infertility tested our relationship to the
limit and strengthened it immeasurably.
Of course we have had our fights. We
grieved together and separately, but I
feel we are stronger for it.*

This man's comment is typical of the many we heard from infertile people. In different words, with different details, they all
told us of the tremendous strain their relationships had endured.
The negative feelings seemed most overwhelming for those who
were still in the midst of the struggle to get pregnant. Those who
had completed their ordeal—who had adopted, were expecting
or already had a child, or had decided to stop trying—expressed
the most positive views. They had a strong sense of having overcome the difficulties.

The experience of infertility profoundly challenges a couple's
relationship. The very survival of a marriage may depend on a
husband and wife's ability to meet this challenge together.

Helen and Dave tried IVF twice and are now waiting with
excitement for a surrogate mother to deliver a baby for them.
Dave described how much their lives had changed since the
simple and carefree times when they were first married:

We were just going along and having a good time. We had
a lot of friends and we were both excited about our work.

When we realized that we might not be able to have a child, everything fell apart. For years after, it seemed like every thought, every word, was focused on what we had to do to get Helen pregnant.

It's very difficult for me to imagine that anything else could happen that would require more of us than what we've been through over these last five years. We found out just how much we need each other. We are a team. Our marriage is strong. We did it!

Helen explains why it was so difficult:

Sometimes I wondered if we were going to get through this as a couple, and sometimes I wondered if I was going to survive at all. The years seemed endless. Sex became a burden, and there were so many procedures, which were painful, tiring and expensive. At times I felt I was going crazy with depression. John tried to be supportive, but from the beginning, the emotional intensity was much less for him than it was for me.

I finally came to understand that he just didn't experience it the way I did, so now I accept that difference. And he tried to understand my feelings—the disappointment, and the guilt I felt for being jealous when friends got pregnant. By the time we made the decision to try in vitro, we had worked out a lot and turned into a pretty good team. I think we will be better parents for it.

Stresses on the Couple

It is the rare couple that experiences infertility without some strain on their relationship. There are many reasons for this stress—the emotional ups and downs from month to month, the financial drain, the distortion of lovemaking into scheduled baby making, and the tremendous physical risks taken by the woman.

The financial demands alone can take their toll, as people give up so many other things they want or need in order to spend their money on physicians and lawyers. Some women quit their jobs to be available for treatments, reducing the family income at a time when expenses are greater. Some people resent the high costs of treatment because getting pregnant seems to be "free" for everyone else. They also become angry at the insurance companies that will not cover their treatment, claiming that it is not medically necessary.

Resentment, anger, and feelings of deprivation can undermine a relationship. The same is true for low self-esteem. Individuals who do not feel good about themselves find it hard to be loving and to be loved in turn. A woman who has undergone AIH unsuccessfully for a year wrote:

> Probably the worse effect infertility has had on our marriage is that it made me an incredibly serious and depressed person. My husband is having a hard time living with this new me—we used to have so much fun together.

For many couples, the dramatic swing from despair to hope and back to despair again is the hardest to deal with. Many people described this as a roller coaster, from which they cannot get off until they are successful.

Once a couple decides to attempt an alternative, they must go through procedures that are often rigorous and demanding. The testing, the timing, the visits to the doctor, the waiting for results all put tremendous stress on a couple attempting to support each other. One social worker at an IVF program said that some couples find the procedure puts too much strain on their relationship, and they quit after one attempt. Other couples may need time away from the program to work out their differences or to seek marriage counseling before trying again.

Infertility is often discovered early in a marriage, before couples have ever needed to work out how to cope with a crisis. Sometimes couples have difficulty knowing how to give each other support. The woman may find her husband preoccupied and unsupportive, and he may be angry and frustrated about not being able to make her feel better or to find a solution to their problem.

Even when anger is not an issue, even when a couple has had a close relationship, they are still two individuals whose responses to infertility are bound to be different from each other. It is impossible for two people to feel the same way at the same time. Grief is a lonely process, and even the most loving partner cannot know all the other's feelings or make the guilt and depression go away. One woman who had been trying to conceive for five years wrote:

> I cried, and my husband couldn't understand why I was so upset, so I cried more! A vicious cycle!

Another woman who has been infertile for ten years told us:

> I try to be understanding, and I do think I understand much
> more now than I did when we first went into this process.
> But I also feel that I don't have a lot of energy left over to
> be real supportive of him. I gotta hold myself together too.
> He's worked very hard to keep his feelings down and I'm
> afraid he's just never going to work through it. But I can't
> do much more; I can't do it for him. He has to handle it his
> own way.

Infertility is not an event that occurs and then slowly recedes
into the past, like most losses. It is an ongoing, recurring loss,
one that forces couples to make many decisions at a time when
their relationship is already strained. They must choose at various times whether to stop or continue. Should they get another
opinion? Can they afford another round of IVF? Is it worth going
for one more test, one more month of Pergonal? Can they live
with having another woman bear their child? Which adoption
agency might give them the quickest results? When they disagree about the best direction to take, they must work hard to
resolve the conflict.

So often these stresses are faced in isolation. Family and
friends often cannot understand or do not know how to be
supportive. Partners are forced to turn to each other for most, if
not all, of their support. It is a heavy burden for them to help
each other while feeling so vulnerable. One man wrote us reflecting on how much better he felt after finally talking with
others who are infertile:

> It has been a painful growing experience. We handled the
> first two years alone, confiding in few people. Only recent-
> ly have we realized how well we had managed an issue that
> many find almost intolerable. Despite many hurting mo-
> ments, we are closer than ever.

Men and Women: Different Responses

There appear to be sharp distinctions between the way most
men and most women react to the crisis of infertility. Many
individuals see the conflicts in their relationship as arising from
their own or their partner's personal failings. Yet there is a com-

mon pattern of male-female differences that often puts further stress on a couple. The way in which men and women cope with their feelings, for instance, tends to be different. Very often the men withdraw while the women prefer to talk. One woman, for example, talked about how busy her husband would become at the difficult times during their struggles with infertility:

The day we heard that the IVF didn't work, my husband threw himself into a community project. He really needed to do that so badly because he is very threatened by my feelings of loss. He can be supportive for a while, but then he always backs away and gets angry when I cry.

One man described his way of dealing with the tension. Instead of withdrawing emotionally, he would try to joke about the situation. He said:

The most difficult part, I think, was supporting her. She was the one who was feeling the most physical and emotional stress. I tried to make it better by being as silly as possible because it was an absolutely absurd situation going through all this stuff. Somehow I knew that silliness was not what she wanted, but it was the only way I could deal with the IVF procedure.

Women are more likely to talk to others about what they are going through. They are more likely to organize and attend support groups. When we placed notices in RESOLVE newsletters asking for people who would share their experiences with us, every one of the eighty-five letters we received was written by a woman.

A woman is also more likely than a man to want to discuss marital conflicts with her spouse. For example, one woman said:

He really doesn't want to talk to me about what we are going through. When we start to talk to each other we end up yelling. We resolved that by talking only very briefly. When I suggested we see a therapist he would say, "I'm a boy, boys don't need this." I think that's his way of backing out. I know he feels terribly guilty because it is his infertility problem. I felt I would go crazy if I didn't talk to someone.

The difference between men's and women's feelings about secrecy can be another particularly difficult source of trouble. This difference is especially hard on a woman who needs to talk but feels she must comply with her husband's wishes to keep their infertility problems a secret. In our research, most couples said they agreed with each other about whether or not to tell others of their experiences. Some couples, however, particularly those who used AID, found this to be a problem. Generally, the men were more likely to want to keep everything secret. A woman whose baby was conceived with AID explained:

> My husband insisted we tell no one about the AID procedure, and that was very hard for me. I felt that, in trying AID, I would be carrying another man's sperm, and if the process worked, I would be living with a "lie" the rest of my life. I finally broke down and told a close friend. It felt like I was releasing an enormous pressure from my mind.

Another couple found secrecy an issue between them when using a surrogate mother. The wife said, "I didn't feel as much a need of confidentiality with the surrogate as my husband felt. He was really worried about any contact with her."

We found only one instance in our research where a woman said she wanted to keep her infertility a secret and her husband disagreed. The husband explained, "My wife felt a need to be more secretive about the treatments. As she was diagnosed as having the infertility, she was more sensitive than I."

In most cases where there is a difference in opinion about infertility issues between husbands and wives, it is the husbands' wishes that prevail. Judith Lorber, a sociologist who specializes in the study of health care and gender issues, writes that in our society men's wishes tend to win out in all areas of decision making around fertility. For instance, she cites a study of childless couples in which it was found that if the husband wanted a child and the wife did not, they usually divorced. But if the wife wanted a child and the husband did not, they tended to stay together and not have children.[1]

Not only do men's opinions usually prevail, but as one social worker remarked, many women said they would cover up for their husbands' infertility, saying that the problem was their own. If they had previously told friends that the infertility was their husband's problem, and then they used AID, they would change the scenario to protect their husbands. A woman who wrote to RESOLVE expressed her bitterness about having to cover up her husband's infertility by letting others think that she was the one with a problem:

I was trying to get away from responding to infertility like a case of "cooties," something you feel compelled to pin on "the other guy." So even though I knew my sexual identity was intact, it felt like a hollow reassurance. I seemed to be the only one who knew this. . . . If everyone else sees you as infertile, it is hard not to react as though you are.[2]

Another woman wrote to RESOLVE about the difficulties she was experiencing because her husband wanted no one to know that he had had a vasectomy during a previous marriage. The cover-up even affected the woman's relationship to her own mother, who felt guilty about her daughter's supposed infertility.[3]

Why are women more likely to cover up for men? According to psychologist Ellen Herrenkohl, "It's more acceptable for a woman to admit to having a problem. When couples come to me for marital counseling and circumstances require that one spouse be identified as the patient, it is almost always the woman who volunteers."

This is particularly true when the problem is infertility since, in males, fertility is often confused with virility. One husband who has a Ph.D. in biochemistry offered an explanation:

Society has sterility and impotence all mixed up. Who should understand the difference between sterility and impotence better than I, but my first reaction to learning I was sterile was that I must be impotent. I should know better, but that was my first thought.

Male infertility may also disrupt the unspoken assumption of the man's dominance in a relationship, giving the woman more power than either of them feels comfortable with. Some wives even say they feel guilty about being "whole" when their husbands are not. There are accounts of women actually ceasing to ovulate when AID treatment begins. Do they feel, whether consciously or unconsciously, that they are supposed to be the ones who are infertile, especially since that is what everyone else assumes? Does her assuming the responsibility for infertility restore the previous state of power between them?

Inequalities

A couple's infertility is further complicated by unavoidable inequalities that add to the male-female differences. Every element of the process—the diagnosis, the treatment, the commitment to keep trying, and in many cases the genetic connection to the child—affects the two people in different ways. Inevitably this imbalance also affects their relationship.

Diagnosis

Most often only one partner in the couple is diagnosed as having the infertility problem. Couples can agree that infertility is not anyone's "fault," but it is difficult to avoid bad feelings on both sides. For many, parenthood is part of their expectation from marriage. It is hard for the fertile person not to resent a partner who has in some sense not lived up to his or her part of this implied pact. The affected spouse, on the other hand, often feels guilty and inadequate, convinced of having deprived his or her spouse and having failed the marriage.

The fertile partner is usually relieved at first not to be responsible. He or she may try to be reassuring. As one man said:

> I kept telling her I still loved her just as much, that I married her for herself and not for the kids she would have.

The inequality of diagnosis often means that partners have to be cautious in how they discuss their situation. They feel they must be gentle with each other, not pushing the partner with the fertility problem to do something he or she is not prepared for. This caution makes decision making more complicated, sometimes leading the fertile partner to resort to subtle pressures. In one study of couples seeking AID, the authors made this interesting observation:

> Most often it is the husband who makes the first suggestion [to try AID], possibly because in the majority of cases the problem is felt to be particularly his. As far as the woman is concerned, she is afraid of hurting him or provoking some unexpected reaction by broaching the subject of AID. . . . [But] we often had the impression that the wife had done everything in her power to persuade the husband to suggest AID.[4]

Commitment

Usually women appear to be the most committed to finding a solution for infertility. It has traditionally been considered a woman's problem, and the woman is defined as the patient. Most women are the activists in pursuing alternatives. They do the work; they make the connections; they undergo the tests and treatments. They are identified as needing children the most. It does not matter that the man's condition may be the reason for infertility—the woman is the one who must get pregnant.

Yet in the background we can often detect the subtle but real pressure by the men. It is the men who most often resist the idea of adoption, who want most to have a genetically related child. It is for the men that many women are pursuing a pregnancy, to have "his" child.

Men and women both usually confirmed the view that women are most involved in seeking treatment. One man who has a child from a surrogate said:

My wife was the one; she was the driving force. Put *force* in capital letters.

Most professionals whom we interviewed agreed that the wife usually appears to be more involved. For example, a psychologist who screens couples for IVF believes that it is often the woman who is pushing to try the method, that the man is just going along. She explained:

These women have a real sense of rage. They feel entitled to motherhood. This by all rights should be theirs, and it kind of excludes the men from the whole process. It's their body; it's their business. IVF is really a rigorous procedure, so the men are on the outside. There's a lot of empathy, but they just can't feel what it's like to go through all that.

The apparently greater commitment of most women fits with the popular idea that women want children most and benefit from them the most. There is another side to this picture however. Many clues point to a more complex explanation for women's greater involvement.

An important clue is to be found in the feminist literature of the past two decades, which has challenged the idea that children are necessary to a woman's fulfillment. Feminist authors have emphasized how much motherhood has been an institution controlled by men for their own benefit. Childbearing has had the purpose of providing heirs for men. For women, having children has meant distress and often death. It has also been used to justify women's low pay and lack of opportunities in the work force. Only by glorifying motherhood, by making a myth of how important it is to women, has it been possible to keep women producing children, even when it is the men who want them and benefit from them the most.[5]

As mothers and as feminists, we know the extraordinary pleasure that children can bring. And feminists have been writing more about the value of mothering for many women.[6] But this recognition does not negate the importance of the idea that women's desire for children and their active pursuit of fertility is at least partly instilled by the values of a male-dominated society.

Some of the women say they are driven only in part by their own desire for a child. Their commitment to finding a solution comes from guilt, from their sense of having failed as women because they cannot provide children *for their husbands.* This notion was expressed by a woman who had turned to a surrogate mother to have a child:

> My main emotion was guilt; I felt really guilty that I couldn't provide him with a biological child. If he had married someone else, he probably could have had biological children. Having a surrogate took care of my guilt because I paid for it from the money I had earned, and now he has his own child.

Some of the apparent differences in enthusiasm are a matter of differences in personal style between most men and women. She is emotional and involved, even obsessed, with the efforts. He is the quiet one, apparently detached. Yet he becomes terribly depressed when she gets her period, and he becomes intensely excited by a success.

A psychologist who works with infertile couples observed:

> The women tend to be more open in general. Some of the men are so controlled, reserved, cautious. Once there is a pregnancy, they just let themselves go, and even their wives are surprised. They just weren't willing to get their hopes up until it was a reality.

Some men told us they feel reluctant to encourage further treatments because they cannot stand to see their wives going through any more tests or suffering any more disappointment. It is not that they want a child any less, but they recognize that it is their wives who must endure the physical and emotional strain of treatment. Usually, then, they do not want to push too hard, agreeing to go along if she really wants to proceed.

When one partner is more committed to seeking a solution than the other—whether it be the man or the woman—this imbalance can cause serious problems. One woman whose husband was ambivalent about having a child described the result:

> I desperately wanted a child, and my husband went along with doing AIH, but he really had a lot of conflicts about it. Asking him to produce a sperm specimen twice a month in the doctor's office became an unbearable chore. He just hated the whole process. We had so many fights, now I can't even tell him when I get my period. I have to hide the little wrappers from the tampons because he gets so depressed.

Treatment

No matter how united a couple is, the man is inevitably a bystander when his wife is trying to get pregnant. At best, he can be supportive. He can take the woman's urine or blood to the lab, sit with her through ultrasounds, wait for her to wake up from laparoscopies, or hold her hand during inseminations. Then comes the one task that only he can do. In the diagnosis stage and for all of the methods except AID, he must produce sperm. He must go into a bathroom in the hospital or doctor's office and masturbate into a cup.

This simple act is not so easy for many men. Women have their most private parts examined and invaded by a host of strangers, over long periods of time, yet the man's solo encounter with himself in the lavatory is fraught with discomfort. Whether because of embarrassment, religious reservations, or a strong overlay of performance anxiety, our interviews were filled with awkward joking about this one aspect of the treatment. A man whose sperm was used to inseminate a surrogate recalled the friendly teasing of his friends:

> There was a point where we thought it might be twins and some of our friends started calling me "megasperm." They would joke around and ask how it feels and I would say, "oh, it's all in the wrist."

For women, resentment may arise from this imbalance in involvement. One woman recalled:

> It was his problem, but they did very little to him. They turned to me and did a whole bunch of tests just to double check if everything was OK. It doesn't seem fair.

Another woman had been through one cycle of IVF and was being encouraged by her husband to try it again. Her response:

> It's easy for a man to say, "Let's do it again"—they don't have to go through it!

Women who go through IVF for male infertility may have the most cause for resentment. After all, they are presumably healthy. Yet they become the patients, undergoing powerful drug treatments, daily ultrasounds, and surgery under general anesthesia in an effort to have "his child."

Many women did not express these feelings. They accepted the difficulties and stress as necessary to achieve their goal. It had to be done, they felt, and would all be worthwhile if they could only have a baby.

Parenting

When deciding to try a new technique that requires using a donor, there are many more issues of inequality for a couple to consider. A social worker at a fertility program explained:

> The most complex component is that one person is the biological parent and the other is not; so they start off on an unequal footing even before the birth of the child. They have to resolve with each other what the meaning of being parents is and the difference between biological and social parenting and how they feel about this inequality in biological parenting.

When couples talked with us about this imbalance, they expressed strong feelings and widely differing opinions. One woman said:

> I would rather do AID and have a donor than adopt—at least it's half of ours.

Other people expressed the opposite point of view. They felt they could not deal with the imbalance. It would create too many problems either for themselves or for the child. One man explained his decision:

> I want it to be our child biologically or not our child biologically, not half. I don't want to feel involved in something where my wife wouldn't be. I'd rather wait for a new technology that might come along while we are still in our childbearing years that would allow us both to be biologically connected.

In many cases, infertility occurs in second marriages. If one partner already has children, and the other one would like to have a child with the new spouse, the imbalance between the two can be painful. A letter in the *RESOLVE Newsletter* describes the strain this can create:

> I resent my stepchildren and the relationship my husband has with "his" children, and I no longer feel like a couple dealing with grieving for the dream child. I feel as if my husband is the person I've always avoided when I felt weak ... the person who has children. ... He can pick up the phone any time and talk with "his" children. I feel very alone.[7]

Several women whose husbands had children from previous marriages wrote to us expressing similar feelings of insecurity, isolation, and resentment. One woman said she just could not believe her husband was as interested in trying to have a child as she was: "No matter what happens, he still has kids. I don't."

Effects of Stress

The stresses of infertility and of the treatments may affect every aspect of a couple's relationship. They may have a profound impact, for example, on a couple's sex life. The physical and emotional strain of treatment, as well as the depression that accompanies failure, often reduces interest in sex. Sex is no longer a spontaneous expression of love and desire; it becomes a planned, charted, and highly charged activity with the goal of conception. Wolf Utian, director of an IVF program, writes that "the fantasied presence of the gynaecologist in the bedroom directing the sexual activity of the couple" can destroy any desire for intimacy.[8]

Utian also observed, as have other researchers, that a couple's problems may lead the husband or wife to have an affair. He concludes that some people may be trying to test their fertility with other partners.

Infertility can affect a sexual relationship in another way. For instance, psychiatrist David Berger studied sixteen men diagnosed as having a very low or absent sperm count and discovered that eleven of them became impotent for several months following the diagnosis.[9]

So many stresses, so many problems. Do they lead to divorce? Occasionally, when the struggle is too difficult. The husband and wife are simply too far apart in their motivation, their commitment, and their feelings, and they cannot find a way to bridge the gap.

Some couples need a therapist to help them resolve their differences. They may need someone to help them communicate the feelings they have been afraid to share—the fears of abandonment, the ambivalence about trying again and again.

For others, going to RESOLVE meetings is a helpful step. One man said:

> I was surprised to see other people in the same situation as us and many having even more problems. I realized other women could be very emotional, just like my wife, and saw how people can help each other.

Success is a strong antidote to stress. Couples who told us that their relationship was in trouble were likely to be still trying to have a child. Those who had succeeded in having a child, whether through adoption or one of the alternative methods, generally felt much better about themselves and about their marriages. People who had reconciled themselves to not having a child also experienced happier relationships.

One woman who adopted a child after a long bout with infertility and pregnancy loss wrote:

> The adoption has reunited us and made us a real family, not two frustrated housemates. I truly believe that the old saw, Children Can't Save a Marriage, is bullshit. Without our daughter, our marriage was headed for the garbage heap. We couldn't have lived together much longer without a child to love.

Children do not always save a marriage. In fact, therapists have observed that some couples that finally do have or adopt a child then break up. The stress has been too much, and the child cannot "solve" the problems that have festered for so long. Sometimes the couple has gotten used to a childless life-style and after so many years cannot adjust to the major changes a child brings. Or the child they dreamed about and worked so hard for may fall short of the perfect baby of their fantasies.

Most couples survive, however, with or without children. They claim that their relationship is stronger than ever, that their partners' love made it possible to survive so much trauma. Many comments from people we interviewed reflected this process of change and growth. As one woman said:

> It may be a cliché to say adversity has strengthened our marriage, but I think it probably has. We went through everything together. We have bonds and trusts that other people don't have. We know how to deal with each other's disappointments and have learned that, despite all our problems, we are very fortunate. We know our children are miracles, and we're so grateful.

10
High-Tech
Children

These are very much wanted children.
These kids, you know, are dropped from
heaven. I wonder how that's going to
affect them.

—Mother of a child conceived through IVF

Will being so special—the "miracle babies" who came after years of infertility—create problems for these children? Perhaps they will not have any special difficulties. It is possible, though, that their parents will overprotect them or worry excessively about their health. Such children may find it hard to live up to everyone's expectations. Perhaps they will be teased by their friends about coming out of a test tube.

When a donor is involved, the repercussions for the children are likely to be even more complicated. How much should they be told? How will they feel about having a "third parent"? Should they have any contact with the donor?

It is not surprising that the parents of "high-tech children" are uncertain about the answers to these questions. No one really knows the long-term effects of the alternative methods. We will not know what they are for many years, since almost all of the hundreds of children born from IVF and surrogate mothers are still very young. We know very little even about the tens of thousands of children born through AID who have already reached adulthood, because of the lack of follow-up studies. We know nothing about the future of OT children, since the procedure is so new and has produced only a few babies. Since there is no information on the potential dangers, these children must be considered part of a massive social experiment for which they have not volunteered.

When prospective parents think about the risks of the new alternatives, however, their immediate concern is with the physical risks—the health of the child—rather than with long-term psychological effects. They fear that egg or sperm donors may harbor unknown diseases, such as AIDS. The idea of conception in a "test tube" arouses fears of mistakes in the laboratory or some scientific mishap. Some prospective parents are concerned that a surrogate may not be taking good care of herself during the pregnancy.

The data that exist so far show that children born of AID and IVF are healthy, although some experts worry about the long-term effects of these methods.[1] There are no studies yet on the health of children born to surrogates, but neither is there any reason to expect that the health of these children will differ from that of other children.

Special Problems for the Children

Once a child is born and appears to be healthy, the parents begin to think more about the psychological issues. With hardly any information to guide them, how are they to know what is best for their child? We do have information about the adoption experience, which, although not the same as the methods discussed in this volume, is concerned with similar issues for the children. Adoption is most similar to the methods involving donors. However, even children born from AIH or IVF and related genetically to both parents may face some of the same problems as adoptees. In most of these situations, the children are part of their families because of their parents' infertility. Their future is very much affected by the parents' ability to resolve this part of their lives comfortably.

A number of researchers have claimed that adoptees exhibit more emotional problems and are more likely to seek therapy than nonadoptees. They attribute this to the fact of adoption. Others disagree on the reason, suggesting that adoptive families may simply be more comfortable asking for professional help. Some psychologists also point out that if adopted children do have more problems, it is probably not because of the adoption itself but because of poor communication in the family. Both parents and children may use adoption as an extra "weapon" in the normal parent-child struggles.[2] Arthur Sorosky, Annette Baran, and Rubin Pannor, authors of *The Adoption Triangle,* agree that the impression of adoptees as having major problems is exaggerated, but they point out that pitfalls do exist:

> Although we would agree ... that it is wrong to blame all the adoptees' problems on the adoption experience, there is evidence to suggest that adopted children have unique areas of vulnerability. Adoptive parents must be acutely aware of their children's special needs.[3]

What are these "unique areas of vulnerability," these "special needs"? One important concern for many adopted children is the feeling that they are not the parents' first choice. Psychologist Ellen Herrenkohl, for instance, says that adoptees with whom she has worked often exhibit an excessive need to please their parents and fear being rejected by them. When there is not a genetic tie to the parent, she explains, the child may feel that it would be possible to "give him or her back," that the connection to the parents is not eternal and unconditional.

Adopted children are often told that they are extra special because they were "chosen." Yet, according to Betty Jean Lifton, author of *Lost and Found,* "chosen baby" stories are more upsetting than reassuring. She writes:

> Many adoptees have told me that the stories made them feel twice rejected; by the natural parents who didn't keep them, and by the adoptive parents who couldn't have a baby of their own. Being *chosen* meant being second best.[4]

The reality is that the parents *would* have greatly preferred to have a child the "normal" way. Adoption, IVF, or AID was not their first choice, but something they turned to when their efforts to conceive failed. This is not necessarily a problem for the child unless the parents have not accepted their infertility and see the child as a constant reminder of failure.

Jerome Smith and Franklin Miroff, authors of *You're Our Child,* comment about their research on adoptive families: "The ease with which the child fully accepts his adoptedness is directly related to the degree of success the adoptive parents have achieved in accepting their own status of adoptive parents." They add that the parents who talk too much or not at all about adoption, who are unable to handle a friend's pregnancy, or who are "struggling with fantasies of how their own biological children might have looked or behaved" will communicate to the child a feeling that something is wrong.[5] These observations apply not only to adoption but to families who have used the new methods of conception as well.

Some parents, for example, form an excessively protective relationship with the child. Having waited so long and being so aware of the preciousness of this child, they cannot let him or her out of their sight. One woman, in a rather extreme situation, tied red ribbons between herself and her daughter and never left her side.

People who have children after so many years of effort often have unrealistic expectations of themselves as parents. They cannot imagine complaining about the daily hassles, for they are going to be perfect parents. This can cause a great deal of strain for them and the child. After all, "miracle babies" spit up and cry at night and have temper tantrums just like any other kids.

The parents may also have unreasonably high expectations of the child. This child, born of science as well as intense devotion, can hardly turn out to be average. Their expectations of children may be even greater with AID, because the donors are chosen from highly intelligent, successful men. The reality is that the child may be much more accomplished than the parents, but unlikely to achieve the level of the most brilliant biological father.

The child may also have impossibly high expectations of him or herself. After all, the parents suffered and worked hard to have him or her. They spent a lot of money, devoted all their energies to becoming parents, and dreamed about the wonderful child they would have. The child may feel that he or she has to be perfect to satisfy the parents.

On the other side, it becomes easy to explain undesirable behavior as coming from "bad blood"—"Surely she couldn't have gotten that from me!" the parent may say. Even normal misbehavior can be construed as a problem, one that was inherited from someone else. When the donor is unknown, such thoughts are more likely to occur.

In most cases of adoption, the child imagines a birth mother who was young and poor and became pregnant carelessly outside of marriage. She could not even take care of her own child. As a result, adoptees often feel ashamed of their origins and, as adolescents, may act out with rebellious and, ironically, promiscuous behavior.[6]

A surrogate mother, in contrast, did not create the child by mistake. She is likely to be married and can be presented as a generous person who wanted to help the parents. Yet questions will certainly still exist in the child's mind. How could she have given him or her away just for money? What kind of cold-blooded person could she be? Not the adoptive child's fantasy of an immoral or poverty-stricken mother, but surely a concern about whether the mother cared more about money than about the child.

A child born of AID reflected a similar feeling about the role of money in her conception, as quoted in a study by Joseph Davis and Dirck Brown:

> I wanted to know how he could have sold what was the essence of my life for $25.00 to a total stranger, then walk away without a second thought. ... Why couldn't he connect the semen to the human being it would create?[7]

Children as well as the parents who raise them often wonder what traits they may have inherited from the donor or birth parent. This opens the door for children and parents to fantasize. One adoptee quoted in *How It Feels to Be Adopted* reminds us that there can be very positive sides to the fantasies:

> The best thing about being adopted is that I can have wonderful fantasies about my birth mother. And if you're a dreamer, which I can be, your mother can become anyone you want her to be. I happen to like opera a lot, so for a while my real mother was Maria Callas. She was such a strange and wonderful lady, and I thought it was neat to have such a bizarre and exotic mother.[8]

A child born from one of the new methods is different from an adoptee in one important way—he or she is usually genetically related to at least one parent. This may be an advantage over adoption, since the child will feel connected to part of his or her family heritage. It may also present problems for the family, however, if it becomes the source of power struggles between the parents. In almost all two-parent families, there is an imbalance of power. It is also normal for children to favor Mom sometimes and Dad other times. The danger in families that have used alternative methods is that common situations will be interpreted as having genetic meaning, creating unnecessary anxieties. One woman who had a child from AID gave an example:

> There are times when I feel my husband is not taking his full share of responsibility for our child. This conflict would probably have arisen no matter what the circumstances of conception, but I wonder sometimes if my husband feels his son is more mine than his.

Many people who are trying to conceive already have one or more children. These children could also have special problems with their parents' infertility. They may feel the anguish of their parents' ordeal, sometimes assuming—as children do—that it is their fault. A woman whose son was six when she started infertility treatments recalled:

> He started having panic attacks, and I was so concerned, I took him to a psychiatrist who helped him verbalize his feelings. It turns out he thought we were angry at him, that it was his fault. He even asked me if giving life to him had ruined me so I could no longer have any more children!

If a sibling does arrive, will the usual rivalry be worse because of the circumstances? Will this very special new child seem to the older sibling to be more wanted, more loved?

Although the parents may feel very comfortable handling any problems that arise within their family, they may still fear that disapproval by others will hurt their children. The popular view assumes that a child is best off with his or her biological parents. Often-heard phrases such as "Blood is thicker than water," "Is she your own?", or "Is that your 'real' mother?" convey this message.

Approximately one in every one hundred Americans was adopted by nonrelatives, and many children live with parents who are not genetically related to them.[9] There is still a "cultural lag," however; most people's values have not caught up with the reality. Our society still holds on to the norm of a "traditional" nuclear family, a norm that may affect the many children who do not fit the ideal model.

In the next few years, however, the number of children born through IVF and the other alternatives will be large enough that a child will not have to feel he or she is the only one. In addition, parents who have become friends through RESOLVE or infertility clinics are likely to bring their children together as they meet to talk through the problems they face and to celebrate the growth of their children.

The Search

Adopted children often report a need to know their origins, to know they weren't "dropped from heaven" or "hatched in a social agency." One thirteen-year-old quoted in *How It Feels to Be Adopted* said:

> Adopted kids ... need to know where they came from, instead of thinking that they just appeared on this earth from outer space ... everyone goes through an identity crisis at one time or another and everyone needs to know where he or she came from. As soon as I searched and found the information I was looking for I felt more worthwhile in the world—as though I belonged better. Beforehand, a part of me had always been missing.[10]

No matter how good adoptive parents (or the parents who have used alternative conceptions) are in relating to their children, the children will always have some normal curiosity about their origins. This interest surfaces at major turning points in their lives, such as during adolescence. It may subside after that, but later life crises often reawaken the yearning for their roots. Marriage, pregnancy and parenting, death of an adoptive parent and the presumed old age and death of the birth parents are all reminders of the adoptees' separation from their genetic heritage.

Many times adoptees who seek information about their origins realize that the parents are uncomfortable with their questions, and they learn it is better not to ask. This lack of openness can only create further problems. One adopted woman quoted in *The Adoption Triangle* talked about this issue:

> I was very curious about my birth parents, but felt that my adoptive parents became angry because I wanted to know

more. They felt they had failed me because of my curiosity.[11]

Questions about origins can be threatening to the adoptive parents. Yet one study suggested that reunions between adoptees and birth parents led to even better relationships with the adoptive parents.[12]

A major theme in the adoption literature is "the search." Adoptees often respond to their need for a biological connection and concerns about identity by looking for the birth mother. This has been extremely difficult, since the laws and adoption agency policies, and sometimes the adoptive parents, put obstacles in their way. Yet the desire for reunion persists on both sides, and the courts and adoption agencies have recently started to pay attention to this need and have considered revising their policies.

It is interesting that female adoptees are more likely to search than males, and mothers are more accepting of a search than fathers. The search is almost always for the birth mother. As in so many other areas of social life, it is the women who are forging the connections that link people together.

We expect that children born to surrogate mothers will also want to find the women who gave birth to them, even though one genetic parent is known. They will engage in a search for the same reasons adoptees do, to know about their origins and to meet the women who carried them and gave them away. They may be at an advantage compared to most adoptees, since the adoptive parents ordinarily have much more information on birth mothers who were surrogates, and no laws require the sealing of records. How easy it will be depends, however, on the wishes of their parents and the policy of the particular surrogate program.

Most surrogate programs act as a go-between for couples and surrogates whenever they want to have information about each other. This service makes possible updates on medical information and can be a way to locate each other at a later date. One program in California requires that changes of address be sent to it by both parties for eighteen years after the birth. There are no guarantees, of course, that this information will be sent to the programs or even that the programs will survive.

Some surrogate mothers may search out the child themselves, as birth mothers of adopted children are doing increasingly. No matter who initiates the search, there is a strong likelihood that many surrogates and the children to whom they gave birth will meet each other. OT donors, in contrast, are much less involved in the child's creation than a surrogate mother. Some want to maintain contact with the children; others consider their donation to be like AID—short term and impersonal.

The likelihood of AID children meeting their genetic fathers is very remote. Even if they do find out about the conception, so few physicians keep records that it is usually impossible to trace the donor. Yet some adults conceived by AID are searching anyway, resorting to medical school yearbooks and attempting to obtain information from the physician. Some American experts have urged that records of at least the donor's characteristics and medical history be kept and made available to the children, but it is unlikely this will happen soon.[13]

When Sorosky and colleagues examined the outcomes of hundreds of reunions between adult adoptees and their birth parents, they were impressed with the intense emotional quality of the search and the benefits of its success:

> For a human being who has been unnaturally separated from his/her origins, the reunion with a birth parent is an integral event in his/her life. ... The reunion provides a bridge to the adoptee's beginnings and answers questions about the past and present. Whether the outcome of the reunion fulfills fantasies is not so important as the fact that it gives the adoptee, finally, a feeling of wholeness.[14]

The Child's Relationship to the Surrogate Mother

Surrogate birth raises the additional dilemma of what kind of relationship the family will have, if any, with the woman who gave birth to this child. Should she be like a favorite aunt who visits on holidays, a close friend of the family, or a more distant figure? What will be best for the parents? What will be best for the children?

One possible model is "open adoption," which has been an important response to the difficult search experiences of so many birth mothers and adoptees. In open adoption, the adoptive couple may meet the birth mother, often prior to the birth, and continue a relationship of some kind after the adoption, or they may correspond with each other through the agency.[15]

Some variations on this approach have been followed by many couples who hired surrogates. In some cases, the adoptive parents and the surrogates have maintained contact, and the children have already met their biological mothers once or several times. This may also occur with donors in the ovum transfer program who will stay in contact with recipient couples.

An ongoing relationship between child and birth parent could be very positive, or it could cause problems. The birth mother or surrogate may be in a position of competing with the adoptive mother for the child's attention, or she may disagree about how the child should be raised. This may be particularly true when the donor parent and the adoptive parent are members of the same family. The adoptive mother is vulnerable to feeling insecure in this situation because she has not given birth to the child.

One father of a boy born to a surrogate told us:

> I suppose eventually he will want to meet her. I don't think you can deny the child that or the biological mother if she wants it. I don't have a problem with that. I just think it could be a little confusing for the kid.

A fifteen-year-old adopted girl quoted by Jill Krementz confirmed that knowing two mothers does have its difficult aspects:

> It's confusing because I don't know how to categorize my relationship with Alison [the birth mother]. I don't want to think of it as purely biological, but I don't know how else to define it. I feel ridiculous introducing her as my friend and yet I certainly don't think of her as my mother. . . . My birth mother's the person who gave me my heredity and my life, and while I don't want to push her away I also don't want to take anything away from my Mom.[16]

In the near future it is certain that a growing proportion of surrogate mothers will have no genetic connection to the child at all. Embryos that grow in the laboratory through IVF are already being transferred to hired women who have been given hormone treatments to prepare them for pregnancy.

The situation where the birth mother acts as "incubator" for the product of other people is still very new, and the consequences for the children are not known. How will they feel about having grown inside a stranger's body, about being borne by a woman who saw herself as only a carrier? Perhaps they will feel less compelled to search for the "host mother" if there is no genetic connection to her. The chances of a relationship will be even smaller than with other surrogate mothers.

There is no one best model for how these complex relationships should work. Every family must resolve the dilemmas in its own way. What is most difficult is that the interests of those involved may conflict with each other. The parents, the donors, and the children may all need, or want, something very different from one another.

Telling the Child

Aware of the possibility of problems, many parents wonder if they should tell a child about his or her origins at all. Their decision depends a great deal on the particular method involved.

For people trying IVF, for instance, secrecy is not much of an issue. Everyone we surveyed who has or is trying to have a child through IVF intends to tell the child. They generally want the children to know how special they are. But they must proceed with some caution, as this mother of an IVF child points out:

I want her to know what we went through so she will understand how special she is to us. But I think you can get into a bind—you don't want it to be something she has to live up to.

Couples who hired surrogates were a little less sure, but they generally planned to treat the subject openly. Surrogate birth is similar to adoption because of the existence of a birth mother who relinquishes the child to a couple through a legal adoptive process. Not surprisingly, most parents expect to tell their children about their birth mother in the same way professionals now advise parents to talk about adoption—gradually, openly, and early in the child's life.

The parents of AID and AIH children, in contrast, are divided and uncertain about what to do. Couples who use AIH may feel that there is no reason to talk about the conception with a child. For couples who use AID, however, telling presents the most difficult dilemma. Of all the alternatives, artificial insemination is the only one that has been treated with so much secrecy. Hardly anyone suggests that other procedures be kept secret. Instead we hear that the child *should* know how much he or she was wanted.

Why the tremendous difference in attitude? The key difference seems to be that artificial insemination usually involves male infertility and that other methods usually treat female infertility. AIH, which can be used for either partner's problem, is more likely to be kept secret when used for male than for female infertility. It appears that the couples, and society as a whole, consider male infertility a much more serious stigma than female infertility. Men judge themselves and are judged by others by their ability to "perform," whether it be at work, in bed, or in producing offspring. A man who is lacking in any one of these domains feels deficient in all areas of life. This can be seen in one father's comments:

> When I told my son about his AID origins, I also said that
> I still have an erection, so he would know that infertility is
> one thing and potency something else.

Infertile mothers rarely feel compelled to explain to their adopted children that they can have orgasms. It appears that secrecy is more for the protection of the husband than for the benefit of the child. This may not even be recognized by the couple, who focus their concerns on what they judge to be the child's welfare.

It is much easier to keep AID secret than other forms of conception, and certainly easier than adoption. There is no legal transaction, and the mother has an apparently normal pregnancy and birth. The father's name is on the birth certificate, and often the attending obstetrician or midwife is unaware of the AID. In addition, most physicians who offer AID and therapists who counsel prospective AID parents strongly advise the couples to maintain secrecy, never to tell the child or anyone else.[17]

The reality, however, is that many children will suspect something and be troubled by their suspicions. Most couples do tell a few friends or family members. In addition, the mother's medical records may include information about AID. The potential for divulging the secret is always present. If they do find out from others, the children will learn that their parents can deceive them about something so central to their identities.

Studies of adopted people suggest that the child's knowledge of his or her origins may indeed create problems, even turmoil. Yet they also show that a lack of complete information and understanding is even more harmful.[18] This is a harsh dilemma for parents who are committed to openness in their families yet fear the consequences of telling. One man wrote to us describing his ambivalent feelings about this question:

> Ideally, I don't want to lie to my child or deceive her by failing to tell her the whole truth. It doesn't seem right for me to decide that she doesn't need to know the truth about her conception. Yet, if I do tell her about it when she's old enough to understand, it could be too upsetting for her. After all, she would never be able to trace the donor if she wanted to. Why cause problems unnecessarily?

Jim is a father who resolved these questions by deciding to tell his son Michael, even though he worried about what the news would do to their relationship. He described to us his reasons for telling his son about AID and the "momentous day" when he did finally share with Michael the story of his conception:

> It was too stressful keeping this information from my boy. I don't think my wife and I ever sat down and said, "We need to tell Michael. When should we tell him?" I think it was understood that it was my job, since I'm not the bio-logical parent.
>
> I knew in his earlier years that he was too young to understand; he didn't have enough information to process what I was going to tell him. But on the other hand, I wasn't going to wait until adolescence, because then, with what-ever else was going on between us, this would just be thrown in the hopper. It would be a terrible betrayal. He's ten now, and I knew it would have to happen soon. I wasn't nervous because I hadn't planned it out; it happened really spontaneously, and I will just never forget it.
>
> I was jogging in the morning and he was riding his bike along with me, and we saw a dog go by and I said, "You know, I'm really afraid of dogs." I told him there was a runner who got his testicle ripped by a dog, and Michael said, "Oh really, can that man still have children?" And I thought, "O.K., he knows, he's got that information." So I said, "Michael, there's something I've got to tell you." And I told him. I was running, and he was riding his bike. He wanted to know whose sperm it was. I said, "We don't

know who it was, but we know that it was a medical student in New York." And we ran on a little bit, and he said, "You know, maybe that's why I want to be a doctor." And my heart leaped, because I thought that he has accepted this information in such a positive way. In a sense he was saying that he accepts the fatherhood of this other person, this abstract kind of thing.

And that's how it happened. He didn't seem shocked. We've mentioned it to each other a few times since. I want to make sure he heard it. I will bring it up, not anything dramatic, from time to time, to make it regular, something reinforced, since I guess he could repress it. He doesn't say much, but he knows that on his father's side that's where he's from.

I just felt so good after, I had not realized how much it took out of me to be keeping it from him. I felt like I had completed something, I had ended a travail. I really felt a burden lifted from me. It may be one thing to say they don't need to know, but it's another to say that you as a parent don't need to share it.

More parents are beginning to share Jim's view about AID. Our study showed that somewhat more people (48 percent) intended to tell their child about AID than not (39 percent). The remaining 13 percent were unsure, hoping to find an answer as the child grew older. Our sample is an unusual one, since most of the people are members of the RESOLVE support organization. They are people who are willing to talk about infertility. But they are likely to represent a growing trend toward more openness about infertility.

Other studies have shown that the great majority of parents do not tell their children about AID. When they have told, it has often been due to special circumstances, such as a later divorce and custody battle or the children facing infertility themselves as adults. An important follow-up study by Robert Snowden, G. D. Mitchell, and E. M. Snowden of English families who had used AID found only a few who had told their offspring of the AID origins, and only as adults. In each case, the mother had wanted her son to know he was not genetically related to his father. The husbands in these families were disabled, immoral, or economic failures, and the mothers' revealing the AID could be seen as an act of hostility. In fact it is likely that AID information, kept secret for so many years, may be revealed in an angry environment. Dissatisfied fathers may blurt out to an unruly child, "You're not mine anyway." Studies of adoptees have also found that many were told in an angry way or at an inappropriate time, with damaging results.[19]

On the other hand, Snowden and colleagues also interviewed adults who had been told of their AID origins. They all said that they had suspected something all along and that the telling had been a relief. They also said they felt especially important, and that their relationship to their father was enhanced by realizing what he had been through.[20]

The difficult task in telling for all parents is to make it seem natural and normal. Parents may emphasize that there are other children born in the same way. As one mother wisely commented, "The way you say it is important. You can convince a child that there is a problem if he has five toes on his foot—if you present it like it's a problem."

Psychiatrist Robert Abramovitz agrees. Speaking at a conference of the American Society of Law and Medicine, he said, "Children can handle almost any kind of information. The issue is not whether or not we tell them, but how we tell them and when we tell them." He urges that children born through AID be told because of the potential harm of family secrets. He suggests that the telling should be a part of good basic sex education:

> Telling a child "I'm not your parent" is harmful. Start with "I'm your parent," and then explain that there is more than one way to become a parent.[21]

Telling children about AID as they learn about sexuality and "the facts of life" is a reasonable approach. It is likely to avoid the confusion of a child told at a very young age and the anger of those who are not told until adolescence or adulthood. Ultimately, however, without good studies on the effects of telling and not telling, every family is left to decide for itself what is best for them.

Single Heterosexual and Gay Parents

The majority of single heterosexual and lesbian women who use AID do not keep the information secret. They would rather that others—and the child—realize that the conception was planned and wanted, not the accidental result of a casual affair. Secrecy, then, is usually not a problem, nor is the issue of genetic inequality between parents. The mothers are not worried about protecting men.

A lesbian mother of an AID baby described the relaxed attitude she intended to take in telling the child.

> I'll tell her the truth. Some women have relationships with men, and some women want to have babies and they don't want to have relations with men. Real basic terminology— the sperm and the egg story is still valid. And she'll know other children whose mothers were inseminated. We have lesbian couple friends who are having babies by insemination. So we can talk about "Johnny was inseminated too."

Many people object to AID for single heterosexual or lesbian women because they believe a child born into such a situation will suffer. Yet such children are more likely to suffer from the attitudes of others than from the family environment. Studies that exist do not show a negative effect on children.

Elaine Bleckman reviewed the studies of one-parent families and concluded that there are so many flaws in the studies' designs that it is impossible to say that children are hurt by single parenthood. If they are, it is likely to be a result of poverty or the child's experiencing the loss of one parent through divorce or death.[22] These problems are much less likely to exist when single women seek out AID.

A positive view has also emerged from studies of children living with a gay parent or parents. These children are apparently no different, nor any more likely to become homosexual, than other children.[23] The reality is that family can have many faces, and no particular structure is inherently unhealthy for children.

The Family

When we asked parents if they feel any differently toward their child because he or she was born from an alternative method, the great majority answered with a resounding no. They often qualified the answers, however. For example, they emphasized that AID children are really *theirs* (often underlined). They also expressed an overwhelming gratitude for the children, as seen in this mother's comment:

I do not feel that a child conceived by IVF is different from any other baby born in this world. However, at his birth we realized how much responsibility we'd taken for his conception and after waiting for him for so long, he certainly is *very* special to us. He certainly can't be taken for granted.

Dutch researcher L. H. Levie asked fathers to describe their feelings about their AID children. Their responses suggest the ambivalence—the satisfaction as well as the regrets—that many men experience:

Fatherhood does not cause me any conflicts, although I do wonder sometimes what the child would have been like if it had been my own. The only thing that troubled me terribly was the idea of failing as a man. . . . This obsession has completely gone now that we have this child. I feel rich![24]

One father told us he had a great deal of difficulty accepting the daughter born of AID, and he sought psychiatric help. At about the same time, the girl became very ill and had to be hospitalized. It took this crisis for the father to realize how much he loved the child and how deep was his emotional commitment to her.

However they deal with the unusual origins of their children, most parents try hard to minimize the effects. They want it to be "no big deal," an incidental piece of information. For some parents, this is not difficult, as seen in one woman's comment:

A child is a child and the outcome is always going to be the same—someone to love and cherish. I never think of her as a product of in vitro. She's simply our daughter.

Because they were conceived in an unusual way, there may be some advantages for the children. For example, the fathers of AID children are more involved in the pregnancy and birth than the average father. This is confirmed by a study carried out in Australia, which found 94 percent of the fathers attending the delivery, considerably higher than average.[25] Wives sometimes make a special effort to involve their husbands in parenting, to make sure they feel part of the child's life.

Despite all of the potential difficulties, the adoption literature is reassuring. The great majority of adoptees are as well adjusted as any comparable group of nonadoptees, and the chances are good that the same will be true of the children born of the alternative technologies. These children are much more likely than most children to be born into a family with educated and well-off parents who want them very much. Their parents are likely to be older and therefore more mature, more confident. And they will have the advantages experienced by only children or those with few siblings.

Although there are risks in being a child who has answered parents' years of anguished prayers, there may be a special dimension to the relationship, as pointed out by a sixteen-year-old adopted girl:

> Mother's Day is a kind of wonderful day in our house—between my mother and myself. We've got a different relationship than most people because I'm adopted. If I do something special for her on that day, it makes her more happy than most mothers since, I guess, there's always a fear on her part that I'm not going to think of her as my mother. But I do, because she's the one who raised me and because she's such a terrific person. I never think of my natural mother on Mother's Day.[26]

One woman who found out she was an AID daughter at the age of twenty-one wrote in the *New York Times:*

> Knowing about my AID origin did nothing to alter my feelings for my family. Instead, I felt grateful for the trouble they had taken to give me life. And they had given me a strong set of roots, a rich and colorful cultural heritage, a sense of being loved.[27]

11
Reactions of Others

It's one thing when people watch Phil Donahue's show and hear about bizarre new ways of making babies. It's another thing when somebody they know walks up to them with his own kid who was born that way. After all is said and done, a child is still a child, and people know with their heart that this couldn't be bad.

—John, father of child born to surrogate mother

There is a great deal of controversy over the new methods of conception. Organized political, medical, and religious groups have taken strong positions for and against these technologies. Friends and relatives of infertile people, as well as the general public, may also object to the methods when they hear about them in the news. Yet, as John said, it is harder for people to disapprove when someone they care about wants so much to have a child.

Responses of Friends and Family

Those who share their struggles and experiences with others are often surprised at the positive reactions. They find people curious, interested, excited for them. Many of those we interviewed said their friends and relatives were very understanding and supportive. One woman said:

> All my friends were very excited when we decided to try IVF. They didn't see this as some weird thing to do. We were afraid to tell my parents until after the baby was born. When we did, my mother said, "You know, after all you've been through, this is certainly a miracle for you. She's all the more special."

One surrogate was worried about telling her grandparents, because they were in their late seventies and she considered them very old-fashioned in their ideas and beliefs. She said:

> When I told my grandmother, she surprised the heck out of me because she said, "Kathy, I think that is the most wonderful thing you could do for somebody." It really floored me there for a minute because it wasn't the reaction that I was expecting at all.

Not everyone is so positive, however. People who are trying to conceive have heard plenty of hurtful reactions. "The world is already overpopulated—you should adopt." "You don't know how lucky you are not having kids." "Adopt and you'll get pregnant." "Just be glad you have one child." A surprising negative reaction sometimes comes from people one might think would be understanding and sympathetic. As one woman said:

> A couple of friends who were infertile and were going through the adoption process were very nasty about our finding a surrogate. I thought they of all people would understand. I think they were very jealous.

When negative comments are made by friends or relatives, the relationship usually changes. As one man said: "When you've had an argument like that with someone, you're never quite the same kind of friends."

It is hard not to be angry with others when they oppose a procedure that looks as though it might help. One man said:

> There is a lot of controversy around, a lot of people with religious and legal ideals of how the world should be, with their own axes to grind, and they are trying to impose them on other people.

It is hard enough to be infertile. It is painful and difficult to choose a new route to pregnancy and go through all the arrangements and procedures. The attitudes of others—the misunderstandings and the disapproval—make it even harder.

Public Responses

When IVF programs first began, there was vocal opposition for a short while from "prolife" groups. They picketed the Norfolk clinic and staged a hunger strike in an Australian clinic. The director of the program at Yale University devoted much of his energy at the beginning to speaking to church groups to try to ease their fears. Now, the programs report, the opposition is less visible. According to Linda Lynch at Norfolk:

> I don't hear that much controversy any more, not like in the beginning. The right-to-life people used to really get on us all the time, but not any more. The Catholic church doesn't recognize it, but the general public must be accepting it.

The general public's attitudes toward the new methods vary tremendously depending on the particular alternative in question. This is seen both in the media response and in public opinion polls.

The media, for example, have been most positive about IVF. Reporters followed the first IVF experiences with the same interest and enthusiasm they give to stories of children receiving organ transplants or premature babies being saved by intensive care nurseries. Photographs of healthy IVF babies and of glowing parents appear regularly in the news and in magazine articles. IVF programs seek out such publicity in their competition for clients.

In contrast, surrogate arrangements have often been sensationalized by the media, treated with distaste and fascination. It is true that surrogate programs also seek publicity as a way to recruit women. But they may endure criticism from the media in the process.

AID is rarely mentioned in the news at all. The program as well as the patients are committed to secrecy, and the method makes it easy to keep it secret. It is also not new and does not involve interesting technology. Until a controversial case arises, the media are apparently not interested.

The public is also most accepting of IVF, as seen in a variety of polls. Even in 1978, when only one baby had been born from the in vitro method, a *Parents* magazine poll of fifteen hundred women found that 85 percent of them would approve of IVF for married couples who could not have children any other way.[1] There have been no comparable national surveys since then, but smaller studies of selected groups show continued support for IVF.

We are only aware of two studies that ask for opinions on all of the alternatives discussed in this book. One is our survey of students at two Pennsylvania colleges. The other is an unpublished study, by psychologist Annette Brodsky and her colleagues, of diverse groups including students, infertile people, and participants at a rally for reproductive rights.[2] These two studies, using different samples, reached the same conclusion: AID, surrogate motherhood, and ovum transfer are all less acceptable to most people than IVF. For example, in our study, 60 percent of the students would use IVF themselves if needed, but only 16 percent would turn to AID and 14 percent to OT if they were the only ways for them to conceive a child.

Surrogate programs are the worst, according to these students—only 8 percent would consider them. The students' opinions are very similar to those of the infertile people we surveyed. For them as well, surrogate programs are the least popular of all alternatives. Of the eighty-five people who responded to our questionnaire, only thirteen had even considered a surrogate as a possibility, and almost every one of them rejected the idea.

The programs that involve a third parent—a donor or a surrogate mother—are the ones that arouse the most disapproval. The greater acceptance of IVF is largely due to the fact that, in most cases, both parents are genetically related to the child. Adoption still receives the highest rating of all alternatives in every survey. There is no scientific intervention in the conception, and the parents are equal in being genetically unrelated to the child.[3]

Psychology Today readers who responded to a survey printed in the magazine also agreed that adoption would be their preferred choice and surrogate motherhood their last option.

Although 84 percent would consider adopting if they could not have children, only 14 percent thought they might try a surrogate. AID and IVF were both approved by 48 percent of the people who wrote in. OT was not included in the study.[4]

The students we surveyed were much more approving of the use of the methods by others who could not conceive than by themselves. Although only 8 percent would use surrogates themselves, for example, 39 percent would approve of others using them. They explained that they did not want to tell other people what they should or should not do.

There are limits to this laissez-faire position, however. There is a strikingly lower approval rate (25 percent) if the methods are used by gay people. In addition, for some people in our sample, these methods are unacceptable under any circumstance. For example, students who call themselves "very religious" and attend religious services often are much more likely than other students to object to anyone using the methods. They were more likely to call the methods "immoral" or "unnatural."

Ultimately, public opposition to alternative methods of conception does not affect people personally as much as their friends' negative comments. It does, however, affect infertile people in an indirect way. Public opinion and organized opposition influence decisions regarding what will be researched, who is eligible for services, and what procedures can be reimbursed by insurance. Public opinion also affects laws governing the status of AID children and the legality of surrogate contracts. A single woman who wants a baby through AID, for example, may have great support from her family, but discovers tremendous obstacles in seeking a facility to help her because fertility centers are afraid of negative publicity. A couple who think they might be helped by IVF are likely to be deterred more by their insurance company's decision not to reimburse their costs than by any negative reaction from their friends.

Reasons for Public Disapproval

Why is there so much disapproval of these methods, especially when a third person is involved? Why does the idea of mixing the sperm and egg of a man and woman who are not married to each other make so many people uneasy? The reasons for opposition have not changed much since 1969, when Lou Harris polled sixteen hundred American adults for *Life* magazine about ideas such as the artificial womb, egg implants, and donor insemination. More than half agreed with statements that the new methods would mean the end of babies born through love, that such methods are against God's will, and that they would encourage promiscuity. Many people in the sample had experienced problems having children and welcomed help for infertility, but at the same time they feared the takeover of the family by science and the potential for creating a superrace. Harris quotes some of the reservations:

We should not mess around with the laws of nature. Someone would have to play God, and who's to decide who is the chosen select?

I think I kind of detest the scientific world. It leaves no room for enjoyment. Don't systematize babies.[5]

These fears have not disappeared since 1969. If anything, they have intensified as the new techniques have become more available and well known, and as particularly wrenching or bizarre stories of specific cases appear in the news.

Part of the negative response is due to ignorance. Although most people have heard of the new methods through the media, they often do not realize what is involved. In a 1978 Gallup poll, for instance, 93 percent said they had heard of IVF, but only 42 percent could describe it correctly.[6] IVF has become much more common since 1978, yet the mistaken ideas persist. One woman told us she heard the strangest remarks after telling everyone at work she had tried IVF but had not gotten pregnant. People still asked if the baby was growing in a test tube in the lab and did they have to change tubes as the baby got larger.

Even the relatively educated group of college students whom we surveyed displayed considerable ignorance about the new methods. The questions that asked for their opinions about each method provided some description. Yet, when asked to explain how the alternatives work, fewer than half of the students answered accurately.

Because people do not always understand the methods, many believe that sexual activity is involved with donor insemination or surrogates. Surrogates are sometimes thought to be prostitutes, and a few men have called surrogate programs asking where these women were that they could sleep with. AID is considered by many people to be adultery.

Ironically, sexual fantasies exist about these methods despite the fact that none of them involves sex. But that fact is precisely the reason for many people's opposition to these alternatives. They see the separation of conception from sex as the beginning of the end of marriage and the family.

As with the controversies over birth control and abortion, the idea that technology would allow reproduction to be placed under human control is frightening to many. People fear that such methods will undermine the traditional basis of the family. There is irony here since those who use the methods are desperately committed to family. They have worked hard at maintaining a marriage under extreme stress. Whether married or not, they have invested tremendous energy in having children, something most people don't even have to think about. As Gary Hodgen of the Norfolk IVF program commented:

> Prolife people do not support this, and yet this is the most prolife thing that you can possibly have. How can they not see the value of giving this little baby, which is just like every other little baby when it's born, to a man and woman who so desperately want it?

As the general public becomes more educated, and as people think about alternatives less in the abstract than in relationship to specific situations, their opposition declines. For example, in 1978, when the first IVF baby, Louise Brown, was born, Harris's survey of fifteen hundred women for *Parents* magazine revealed a 49 percent approval of IVF in general. After the procedure was explained, however, and the women were asked if it should be available to married couples who could not have children otherwise, approval rose to 85 percent.[7]

Another reason for negative attitudes toward these methods, besides lack of knowledge about them, is seen in the attitude that considers infertility a minor problem. "It's not a major disease," people say, "It's not going to kill you."

A common reaction is that if a woman cannot have children, then she was not meant to, and it is wrong to try to change that. Some believe, wrongly, that relaxation or adoption will solve infertility and cannot understand why a couple would waste their time with doctors.

People who do not understand infertility or who believe it just could not happen to them seem to be less sympathetic to alternatives. We were surprised, for example, to see that the female students in our study were less likely to approve of each of the alternative methods than the males; females particularly opposed surrogates and embryo transfer. When asked, the students explained that the women are more idealistic than the men, that they have grown up thinking about having their own babies and still hold on to that idea. Their problem was not so much with technology per se, but with the idea of relying on another woman's egg or body in order to have a child.

These are young people, of course, and they have never had to face the reality of infertility. A study that appeared in the *Journal of Social Psychology* in 1977 and included both married and unmarried students found the married women (who were also older) more accepting of alternative methods than unmarried women.[8]

Many of the young women will one day, unfortunately, experience the shock of learning they cannot have babies. At that point, if they are like many of the women whom we interviewed, they will probably feel very differently. They will have a long difficult path, a great deal to think about, as they move from their earlier idealism to the later reality.

Groups in Opposition

The most committed opposition to the new reproductive technologies comes from the Catholic church, fundamentalist Christians, and some representatives of Orthodox Judaism. Surprisingly, some feminists are equally fervent in their opposition to these alternatives. The religious Right and the feminist Left are an unlikely partnership. Yet these groups, which disagree on just about everything else, have found some common ground in their objections to the alternatives for having babies.[9]

Their reasons are very different. For the religious groups, most or all of the alternatives are "moral abominations," violating the sacred marital relationship. As Theodore Hall, a Catholic theologian, wrote, "The child's existence does not justify morally evil means or techniques used in its origin." Some feminists, on the other hand, see artificial reproduction as a means for male control over women's lives and believe it will ultimately be used to exploit all women.[10]

Both groups acknowledge that the children conceived by these methods can bring great happiness to their parents, but they conclude that the drawbacks involved are just too great. For entirely different—indeed contradictory—reasons, they would agree to banning these methods.

The religious objections focus on both the techniques and the possible negative consequences for families. According to Hall:

> Masturbatory methods of obtaining semen must be outrightly condemned as objectively immoral, since it is the church's official, constant (and therefore irreversible) teaching that such acts are "intrinsically and seriously disordered."[11]

Since all the methods require masturbation to obtain semen, this alone is enough to make them unacceptable to the Catholic church and to many Catholics. In addition, the church condemns any procreation that is not a result of sexual relations within a marriage. For example, a surrogate spoke of her cousin who is a devout Catholic who said to her, "It's morally wrong. First of all the masturbation is wrong, the artificial insemination is wrong, giving the baby away is wrong."

Not all religious leaders agree with this position. Orthodox Jewish leaders, for instance, find no basis in Jewish law for opposing AIH or IVF, but most of them object to AID and surrogate mothers. More liberal Jewish and Protestant groups have not taken an official stand against the methods, although individual leaders may find some of them ethically questionable. For example, the World Council of Churches does not object to IVF but would prefer to see the money spent on prevention and cure of blocked tubes and on meeting the health needs of the poor.[12]

Protestant theologians differ widely in their views. Jack Moore, professor emeritus of philosophy and religion at North Carolina Wesleyan College, outlines two major views of theology, one in which humans must not tamper with God's creation, the other in which people are partners with God in improving nature. Those who endorse the second view, he says, are more likely to see the alternatives as acceptable for couples seeking to overcome infertility.[13]

One minister told us of his own ambivalence when first asked for advice, and then the change in his views:

> A couple came to me to talk about their plan to hire a surrogate mother to have a baby for them. They explained how much they wanted to have a family and that it was their only option. I can't say I was happy about the idea, but I also felt I was not in a position to judge them or to tell them not to do this. Now, when I see them with the results—a gorgeous little boy—I am totally delighted.

Not all feminists oppose the methods either. Even among those who see grave dangers in the new alternatives, there are many who are torn by sympathy for infertile women and men, or who would defend the right of single women, heterosexual and lesbian, to have children without sexual involvement with a man.

Ethicists and legal experts offer widely varying views, from full acceptance to total rejection. An important concern that emerges from their many discussions is the "slippery slope" problem—the idea that one action may open the door to others that will be much worse. They wonder, for instance, if technologies that currently are designed to help the infertile will ultimately lead to life being treated as a commodity. Attorney George Annas, speaking at a conference of the American Society of Law and Medicine, vividly described one scenario for the future. He worried that we will one day soon have embryo stores, with catalogs describing the sex, characteristics, and merits of each embryo offered for sale.[14]

Some authors also worry that the possibility of combining IVF with a surrogate mother will lead wealthy women to hire poor women to carry a couple's embryo for convenience. Motherhood would be degraded to a totally commercial activity.[15]

Coping with Disapproval

There is no doubt that the new technologies raise serious concerns about the future of parenthood. For people struggling with infertility, however, the desire to conceive and bear a child often overrides any concern for the objections of others. On the other hand, ignoring one's church or going against public opinion and the attitudes of family and peers may be difficult and troubling. Choosing an alternative often means having to deal with being "deviant," doing something unusual and not always approved of.[16]

The people who try the alternatives have a number of strategies for coping with their "deviance." Some try to educate the public or their friends to change their minds; others resort to secrecy. For some, the idea of being different and doing something unusual has its own attraction. On the other hand, some people have become so used to the insensitivity of others to their infertility that they have already developed thick skins, screening out negative comments. They already know who understands and who will object, and they may choose their friends and tailor their conversations accordingly. As one man said, "Some people are really negative, but we just say 'the hell with them.'"

Some who become involved with alternatives respond to the objections of others by trying to change their opinions with information. The director of the Norfolk IVF program even went to the Vatican to try to influence the Catholic church's position. On a more personal level, a woman who had recently applied to be a surrogate told us:

> I was so excited, I told my friends what I was doing. Then someone would say, "How much money are you getting for that," and I'd get mad and say, "What do you mean how much money am I getting?" That's not the important thing. They didn't understand at first, but when I finished with them they understood and were supportive.

Some take their educational efforts beyond their immediate acquaintances. They go on television shows, speak to reporters, or write up their experiences for magazine articles. They may enjoy the excitement of the publicity, but they also want the public to understand what they are doing. They hope that, by presenting their experiences, they will be able to lessen the opposition. One man reported:

> This might come off real corny, but we're a reasonably intelligent couple and we want to portray surrogate mothering for all the benefits and all the positive things that it's done. That's why we agreed to do the media thing.

Many people wrote us at length about their experiences because they wanted to communicate their views and feelings to the public. Their plea was voiced by one woman who ended a long letter with, "Please tell people about us!"

Total secrecy—not telling anyone what they are doing—is the opposite strategy employed by some of those who are concerned with the negative views of others. It is used most often by those who try AID and sometimes by people involved with surrogates. Some couples who hire surrogates either fake a pregnancy or tell friends that they adopted the child. One woman explained why she and her husband told no one:

> We live in a rural area and people have very, very, conservative values, not necessarily consistent with our own, and it's not our desire to be on the front page of a two-bit newspaper. We don't want our child talked about or teased by the other kids. We knew we were doing something different and some people might frown upon it.

When we requested through RESOLVE newsletters that people who had tried the alternatives contact us, we discovered a striking difference between letters from women who had used AID and everyone else. Many of the AID letters mentioned the desire for secrecy—"Please leave a discreet message when you call," "Please don't use our names," "My husband doesn't want to discuss this." RESOLVE has even set up a separate information network just for AID which allows people to exchange letters with each other in total anonymity.

Associating with other infertile people, especially through RESOLVE, is a helpful strategy for many. A woman who tried AID said:

> It's not something we discuss with the man on the street or with casual acquaintances. In fact, we didn't even tell our family. But we have talked about it with a few people from our RESOLVE group who have become our closest friends now.

Many people who turn to these methods are unaware of the objections or simply unconcerned. Most ignore the religious prohibitions and do not think about what they are doing as related to male exploitation of women. They are not worried about cloning or artificial wombs or any of the visions of the future. They are not looking for an easy way to avoid pregnancy. In fact, they would much rather have a natural pregnancy. All they want is a baby, a healthy baby as close to them genetically as possible. As one woman said:

> I think all the controversies are media hype, because when you are in the middle of it—all you want is a baby and all that other stuff is just superfluous; it really is.

Most people, both providers and their clients, told us that the ethical and legal controversies surrounding reproductive technologies simply do not affect them. They find it hard to believe that anyone could object to what they are doing.

Some people who consider using the alternatives are devoutly religious, yet they often make their decisions without consulting religious authorities. For example, an Orthodox Jewish man whose wife was artificially inseminated with a donor's sperm (a method opposed by most Orthodox rabbis) commented, "I never asked the rabbi if it was OK or not. I guess I just didn't want to hear what his answer might be." A Catholic woman who tried IVF said, "I never talked to my priest about it. The way I figured, it was none of his business."

By avoiding the people who are likely to disapprove and explaining their situation to others who might be sympathetic, most people manage not to hear many open objections. One man said he believes a lot of people are against his hiring a surrogate, but they do not voice their opinion directly to him: "I think if people think it is kind of strange and awkward, they just don't say anything."

There is another reason most people do not respond negatively, despite the reservations they may have. It may be easy to discuss the dangers and problems of these methods in theory, but it is another matter to object to the creation of a real family. For others, just as for the parents, when they see and come to love the children, they are no longer test-tube babies or AID children, they are simply "our kids," "Joe's baby," "Cousin Tammy." This idea was expressed by a respondent in the *Life* poll fifteen years ago: "When you hold a baby who depends on you in your arms, you don't worry where the egg came from."[17]

Conclusion:
An Assessment

In 1977 Russell Baker wrote in his *New York Times* column:

> Until a few years ago, people just happened. As a result, most of them were hodgepodges, like London and Rome, which also just happened.
>
> Occasionally you might run into somebody who had been planned, like Washington, D.C. These planned people were the product of Planned Parenthood. Their parents had sat down with architects. The architects had shown them blueprints of beautiful families in which all the siblings would be as neatly spaced as the oaks on a Washington boulevard. ...
>
> It would be interesting to know what it feels like to be a fully planned person. Having your sex determined by your parents, of course, is surely only a primitive beginning on the intricate architecture which biology will make possible in another generation or so. Before the century is out, science will probably enable parents to decide not only what size and shape their productions will take, but also how bright they will be and what careers they will pursue.[1]

This vision is already closer to reality than even Baker could have imagined at the time he wrote this column. The methods for conceiving that we have described in this book are just the beginning. Scientists are already working on variations that will make it more and more possible to create human beings to the designer's specifications in a laboratory. The changes this will create, for women, for men, for children, for society as a whole, are frightening for us to consider.

Yet we have also felt the agony of those who want to have children and cannot. For them we want the new technologies to work. We want the procedures to be easier, safer, cheaper, and more successful. We want the procedures to be able to help poor women, who are most likely to be affected by infertility but who have almost no access to treatment. We do not want more grief and desperation for people who feel deprived of the chance to be parents.

We are still troubled, however. Our research into the personal experiences of people who consider or try the new methods has uncovered a great deal of trauma and uncertainty. We are troubled by the personal dilemmas, the emotional upheavals, the physical risks, the lack of control, and the unanswered questions about long-term effects.

We are also troubled by the growing role of profit making in baby making. No one should make a great deal of money from the anguish and desperation of infertile couples and from the financial and emotional neediness of donor women. When powerful men and women, whether they be lawyers, doctors, or financiers, make large profits from linking two vulnerable women, we must worry about the consequences.

There is more. Thoughtful observers remind us of past medical discoveries that were supposed to be good for women. DES (diethylstilbestrol) was offered to pregnant women as a cure for miscarriages, a guarantee of healthier pregnancies. Instead it led to cancer and infertility problems for many of their children. The Dalkon shield IUD was inserted in millions of women to give them control over conception. Instead it contributed to massive infections, infertility, and even death for untold numbers of these women.[2]

These are only two examples of products that were heavily marketed to physicians and the public without adequate testing, even after proof of their harmfulness was established. Given this history in the field of obstetrics, many women are asking, "Why should we trust that newer technologies will be any more safe or beneficial?"

Biologist Ruth Hubbard also worries about the long-term effects of interfering with natural reproductive processes by using a technique such as IVF:

After all, embryonic development is the most complicated of biological processes, one in which an infinite number of reactions are taking place in intricate interrelationships, where timing and all kinds of factors in the chemical environment are fantastically important and split seconds or tiny changes in concentration can make a difference. So, coming from this perspective I frankly view with incredibility and horror the notion that one can "simply" remove an egg from a woman's ovary, put it in a culture medium in a dish, and then "simply" pick it up and re-insert it in a uterus that is at the proper stage of preparedness, and have it implant and go through development, without these many manipulations having some effect on the process of development. I cannot believe that there is no effect.[3]

It will be many years before the risks of these methods become known. In the meantime, women and children are once again the guinea pigs in a massive, and potentially dangerous, experiment.

Scenarios for the Future

Hubbard and other commentators are worried not only about the possible physical damage. They also see the shift of conception into the laboratory as another step toward male control over the conditions of motherhood. It is the fear of what may happen with the use of these methods that is most troubling.

It is possible that not so far in the future a young woman will make a trip to the bank after graduating from high school. She will not be depositing her graduation checks, but rather some of her own eggs. In the bank they will be frozen, presumably protected from any future exposure to hazards in the air or at work. She can now be sterilized and never have to worry again about the dangers and uncertainty of birth control. When she is ready to become a mother, she can return to the bank for a withdrawal. A few eggs will be thawed and mixed with the semen (also newly thawed) of her husband, lover, or donor. Scientists will inspect the embryos for genetic defects and for the child's sex. They will look for the characteristics most desired by the parents and add them if they are missing. The future mother can then choose which embryo she or a surrogate mother or the artificial womb will receive to start growing this "ideal" baby.

Some people are horrified by such a scenario. It turns over control of the creation of babies into the hands of the scientists. It makes imperfection, however that is defined, unacceptable. Yet we have described such a scene to women, and they have responded laughingly that much of it sounds very attractive. "Wouldn't that be wonderful if it really worked?" they say. "No worries about birth control, no worries about waiting too long to get pregnant and then being infertile, no worries about genetic defects. We wouldn't have to finish childbearing by age forty. We could really control when and if we want to have children."

Some feminists such as Shulamith Firestone have claimed that women will be truly liberated only when they are free of pregnancy, when completely artificial reproduction is developed in a postrevolutionary society.[4] Freedom from pregnancy, both wanted and unwanted, does have its appeal for many women, especially if they can still become parents.

Many feminists today fear that such liberation will ultimately become enslaving. Once professionals control the "banks" and the technology for conception, they will also be able to dictate the terms. They will decide whose genes should be reproduced, what defects are unacceptable, which embryos should be discarded. In Huxley's *Brave New World,* among the most powerful members of society are the ones who make such decisions, the "Directors of Hatcheries and Conditioning."[5]

Social class will be more important than ever, as poor women are hired to carry embryos for the rich under carefully controlled conditions. Sociologist Barbara Katz Rothman described to us her fear of how this will work:

> I'm convinced that there will be "farms" for surrogates. Once it's possible to implant an embryo created from a man's sperm and a woman's egg into another woman, third world and poor women will be hired for a low fee and kept on the farms to produce highly valued white babies. These women will be carefully watched to make sure they eat right and don't smoke, and people will say it's good for them.

Gena Corea, author of *The Mother Machine,* calls such farms "breeding brothels." She reminds us that control over women—such as black slave women—for use as breeders of children or wet nurses for the wealthy is nothing new in our society.[6]

The most extreme version of such scenarios appears so far in novels such as Huxley's *Brave New World* or Margaret Atwood's

The Handmaid's Tale. In these fictional accounts, reproduction is rigidly controlled by totalitarian rulers in order to perpetuate caste divisions in society. Even these visions, however, are not totally divorced from reality. The Nazis, Corea writes, kidnaped young girls, branded them, and gave them hormones, with the intention that they breed Aryan children and then be killed.[7]

Of course it doesn't *have* to go that far. Most professionals who work in IVF and surrogate programs insist that they are interested only in helping infertile people, not in changing the way everyone reproduces. "Just because you wouldn't want to use a hammer to kill someone," they say, "doesn't mean you should abolish hammers and lose their benefits."

This is a compelling argument. But the question remains: who decides which benefits are worth preserving? For now it is primarily the scientists, for whom the excitement of the research and the prestige of breaking through new scientific frontiers are the foremost goals. They are looking for ways to gain greater control over reproduction in general and ultimately to cure diseases in adults. Through genetic engineering, tissue grafts from embryos, and other experiments, a whole host of other "problems" will be "solved." Some scientists envision the creation of embryos solely for their use in harvesting tissues or organs, a sort of "spare parts" resource. Many infertility specialists agree with the director of Columbia University's IVF program when she speaks of responsible scientists who "live in fear of abuse of the new technology."[8] Yet, as physician Kurt Hirschhorn wrote, "It is a general rule that whatever is scientifically feasible will be attempted." Whatever happened to the idea of these methods being developed for the sake of infertile people?[9]

The scientists and entrepreneurs are cautious not to move faster than public opinion permits. They are carefully attuned to what will be acceptable to most people, at the same time offering new options that stretch the limits of acceptability. They are ready to take advantage of society's growing willingness to allow interventions in reproduction. As James Twerdahl, chief executive officer of Fertility and Genetics Research, told us about the embryo transfer program:

> We will never do it for eugenics or sex selection. The smart clinics will follow trends, not lead them; but, if in twenty

years society says eugenics is good, then we might consider it. If society decides it wants diagnosis of embryos, then we have the delivery system that can do it.

We know that medical products can create new uses and needs where none existed before. As competition grows and products are perfected, new markets must be found. For example, technologies such as fetal monitoring, developed for high-risk deliveries, moved quickly to routine use in almost all deliveries, where they are often unnecessary and may actually cause problems.[10] The wide dissemination of new technologies is often justified on the grounds of patient demand for them. Yet as Corea aptly points out:

> A pattern emerges in the development of many new reproductive technologies. . . . Experimentation on women is presented through the media as a "medical breakthrough." There is much hoopla and many cries of "new hope for the infertile." Infertile women begin clamoring for what they think of as a "new" rather than "experimental" procedure. The demand for the procedure created by the researchers through the media is then used to justify further experimentation on women.[11]

In less than a decade, IVF expanded from being a treatment only for women with blocked Fallopian tubes to being the "solution" for endometriosis, low sperm count, poor cervical mucus, and unexplained infertility as well. What will the next decade bring? Certainly more and more people will be defined as "needing" these technologies. Older women (maybe even over thirty-five), overweight women, women who are working, women who have had cesareans, women under stress, women on medications, smokers, will all certainly "need" surrogates to carry their embryos—created through IVF—in a healthier "environment." We will be told that it is better to have a controlled setting, a supervised surrogate or ultimately an artificial womb.

As sociologist Barbara Katz Rothman points out, all of the new choices offered to women in the area of reproduction can be limiting as well as liberating. A woman does not have a free choice to use a technology if a physician tells her that it is for the good of her baby and she would be irresponsible not to use it. It will not be a choice whether or not to have our embryos or fetuses checked for abnormalities if society condemns women as negligent if they give birth to handicapped children.

In the past, some employers convinced women to be sterilized before they could work in a hazardous setting, but many women resisted.[12] New technologies will be used to overcome the reluctance. Someday soon companies may require prospective women workers to have eggs retrieved and stored, and then be sterilized before they will be hired. Rather than make the work environment safe, they could protect themselves against possible law suits brought by children born with birth defects and by women deprived of fertility.

Infertile people who do not want to endure further procedures can now beg off on the grounds of cost, risk, distance, or their experimental nature. But the programs are quickly becoming more accessible, more routine, and less invasive. Insurance is covering more of the costs. It will be increasingly difficult to say no to IVF and related technologies.

Many of the elements of the futuristic vision are already with us. Surrogates are already carrying embryos that are unrelated to them, and one court has already ruled that such a woman is not legally the mother of the baby she has carried for nine months. Eggs and embryos are being frozen and stored. IVF and sex selection clinics exist in franchise operations all over the world.

Perhaps the greatest fear many people have about sex selection is that the overwhelming preference for sons will be translated into practice. Boys will be preferred, especially as firstborns, and the consequences for girls and women may be disastrous.[13]

Another type of selection—for intelligence—is already going on with donor insemination. In 1982, the first two children were born to mothers who were inseminated with sperm from the Repository for Germinal Choice in California, better known as the Nobel sperm bank. Although not all donors are Nobel Prize winners, they must be exceptionally accomplished scientists— outstanding artists are not acceptable. The purpose of the repository is to "breed more intelligent human beings," as stated by its medical director in a letter to the *New York Times.*[14]

This Nobel sperm bank has been widely criticized for its philosophy. What is usually not recognized, however, is that almost all AID is based on some form of selection, and intelligence is a key criterion. Physicians claim that they usually select residents because they are most accessible, but there are certainly other men who work in hospitals who are not approached. Sperm banks turn away 80 percent of donor applicants, and one of their criterion is university education. At least one sperm bank includes the donor's grade point averages in the profiles they send physicians, and the preference for *A* students is obvious.

What Should Be Done?

Because the present and future dangers of the new methods can be so frightening, many opponents urge that we just stop using them. But what about the legitimate needs of infertile people? Is it fair to deprive them of the technology that might help them have children?

Some writers, such as biologist Ruth Hubbard, respond that the need for children is socially created. It would be better if infertile women overcame the social pressures to have children. She says that some good consciousness-raising to understand that society wants women to think their primary role is breeder of children would be more beneficial than risky technological interventions.[15]

Others add that there are plenty of children available who could be adopted. Since many of these children are members of minority groups, the infertile are accused of racism for not wanting them.

Yes, women need to understand the pressures and to realize that we have other fulfilling roles to play besides that of mother. Childlessness needs to be a much more acceptable solution.

We believe it is unfair, however, to tell infertile people that they must raise their consciousness or overcome their racism in order to give up the goal of having their genetic child or one that would come close. We all need to have our consciousness raised, and we all need to eliminate racism. There is no logical reason that the infertile, who have already suffered social stigma and personal loss, should have to bear these important burdens more than others. Were they somehow designated, because of their biological handicap, to be more virtuous, more selfless, more liberated than the rest of us who can bear genetic children?

Because women have been and are oppressed through motherhood does not make motherhood in itself necessarily oppressive. To want to raise children who do not suffer handicaps, who have not been given up by a grieving birth mother, who bear some resemblance to oneself, who will not have to struggle with the difficulties of being a different race from their parents—for a white couple to desire a healthy white infant is not necessarily racism.

Being a parent is an extraordinarily difficult job under any circumstances, and much more difficult if the child is handicapped, more complicated if the child is from a different racial background. These "special needs children" need to be adopted by especially committed and capable parents. Infertility is not a qualification for being such a parent.

Having a child may not be a right, as some argue. It may not be an entitlement that comes with citizenship, that should be provided by society. Yet to create life, to see oneself in one's children, is to participate in a miracle. It is this miracle that so many people are trying for, one that new technology makes possible for some of them.

For this reason it is imperative that controls be exercised over the use of the technology. Gena Corea proposes a federal regulatory agency on the model of the Environmental Protection Agency.[16] Although such agencies are notoriously poor at regulating industry effectively, often being controlled by the industries themselves, some systematic review may be better than what exists today, which is essentially nothing. Other countries, such as Great Britain and Australia, have established national panels to set policy with regard to reproductive technology. Thus far the United States has done very little, leaving decisions almost entirely up to the practitioners and scientists.[17]

If such bodies are established, it is clearly essential that they not be controlled by the scientists. Their priorities and concerns are different from those of the women and the society affected most by these decisions. Those who make the decisions should include infertile people and representatives from the women's health movement, which has done so much to monitor the effects of medical decisions on women.

◆　◆　◆　◆　◆

Between us we have four young daughters. In fifteen or more years, they will probably be thinking about becoming mothers. We worry about the kinds of pressures and technologies that will shape their choices, or how much choice they will have at all.

What will it be like to become grandmothers then? Will we visit our grandchildren embryos in laboratories and watch them developing as fetuses in their artificial wombs from behind a window, as many grandparents now get their first glimpse of newborns?

Will our daughters be able to accept any hint of imperfection? Will they feel they have to make sure they have a boy first and then a girl, further increasing the male advantage by adding the advantage of being firstborn? Will they select only children who are clones of Barbie and Ken dolls, or whatever the ideal model is at the time?

As we worry about the future, we take comfort from the awareness that people can and do resist the pressures of science and medicine. Women have organized to promote more natural births and succeeded in making very important changes in childbirth practices. Consumer pressures have led to the removal of dangerous drugs and products from the market. Many women refused to believe that formula was really healthier for babies, and they succeeded in convincing mothers and pediatricians alike of the value of breast-feeding. And despite all the surveys and predictions, directors of sex-selection clinics report that couples are much more likely to ask for girls than for boys.[18]

With all of the dramatic social changes of the last decades, almost all women and men still prefer to make babies the "old-fashioned" way. We can hope that better prevention of infertility and better treatments will allow infertile people to do just that, reducing the need for these other methods. And we hope as well that an active informed public will resist the pressures toward conformity and control. We hope our daughters will cherish their individuality and fight for the right to maintain it.

Glossary

AIDS (Acquired Immune Deficiency Syndrome). A fatal disease affecting the immune system, which can be transmitted through sexual contact.

Amniocentesis. A procedure for removing a sample of amniotic fluid from the uterus by inserting a needle through the mother's abdominal wall in order to obtain information about the fetus.

Artificial Insemination (AI). The mechanical insertion of semen into the vagina in order to fertilize an egg.

Artificial Insemination by Donor (AID). The mechanical insertion of semen from a man who is not the husband of the woman whose egg is being fertilized by this procedure.

Artificial Insemination by Husband (AIH). The mechanical insertion of semen from the husband into the vagina or uterus of his wife in order to achieve a pregnancy.

Artificial Womb. A place for a fetus to grow other than a female human uterus.

Blastocyst. An early stage of embryonic development.

Cervical Mucus. Secretions produced by the cervix.

Cervix. The lower section of the uterus, which protudes into the vagina and dilates during labor to allow the passage of an infant.

Cesarean Section. The surgical removal of a fetus by means of an incision through the abdominal wall and into the uterus.

Chemical Pregnancy. A very short-lived pregnancy detectable only through blood tests.

Chorionic Villus Sampling. A prenatal diagnostic test that examines the preplacental tissue for abnormalities.

Cycle. A period of physiological changes occurring between two menstruations.

Dalkon Shield IUD. Intrauterine contraceptive device, now off the market, which contributed to serious pelvic infections in many women.

DES (Diethylstilbestrol). Synthetic estrogen used sometimes as a "morning-after" pill, formerly thought to prevent miscarriage.

Ectopic Pregnancy. A pregnancy that occurs outside the uterine cavity.

Egg Donation. The removal of an ovum from one woman for use by another woman.

Ejaculate. The fluid containing sperm that is discharged from a man's penis during orgasm.

Embryo. The term used to describe the early stages of fetal growth.

Embryo Transfer (ET). The insertion of an embryo into a woman's uterus.

Endometriosis. A condition characterized by pieces of the uterine lining locating themselves anywhere outside uterine cavity. It may prevent conception.

Eugenics. The control of mating to achieve an improvement in the hereditary characteristics of a group.

Fallopian Tube. The tube that carries the egg from the ovary to the uterus.

Follicle. The sac in which an egg develops in the ovary.

GIFT (Gamete Intrafallopian Transfer). A procedure in which eggs are retrieved from a woman, mixed with sperm, and returned immediately to the fallopian tube.

Human Chorionic Gonadotropin (HCG). A hormone that triggers the maturation and release of the eggs from the follicles.

Impotence. The inability to have or maintain an erection of the penis.

Infertility. The inability to conceive or carry a baby to term after one year of sexual intercourse without the use of contraception.

Intrauterine Device (IUD). A birth control device inserted in the uterus.

Intrauterine Insemination. The mechanical insertion of semen into the uterus through the cervix.

In Vitro Fertilization (IVF). A procedure in which eggs are removed from a woman and mixed with sperm in a petri dish. After two days the fertilized eggs are inserted back into the woman's uterus.

Karyotype. The arrangement of chromosomes, including their number, size, and shape.

Laparoscopy. Surgical procedure for visualizing the ovaries and fallopian tubes; used in IVF for removal of ova.

Lavage. Washing out; procedure used in ovum transfer method to remove embryo from donor woman.

Microcephaly. Abnormal smallness of head.

Motility. Ability to move spontaneously.

Motrin. Brand name of a drug used to reduce pain.

Ovulation. The release of an egg from a follicle on the ovary.

Ovum (plural, *ova*). Female reproductive cell.

Ovum Transfer (OT). A new method for infertile women that involves insemination of a donor woman, lavage of her uterus, and insertion of a recovered embryo into the uterus of an infertile woman.

Pergonal. The brand name of a fertility drug that stimulates the development of ova.

Petri Dish. A small shallow container used in a laboratory.

Premature Birth. The birth of an infant before thirty-seven weeks of gestation.

Secondary Infertility. The inability to conceive or carry a baby to term after one or more prior pregnancies.

Semen. A thick whitish fluid produced in the reproductive organs of men and ordinarily containing sperm cells.

Sperm. A mature male germ cell.

Sperm Bank. A place where sperm is frozen and stored for future artificial inseminations.

Stillbirth. Death before birth of a fetus that is at least twenty weeks of gestation.

Surrogate Mother. A woman who agrees prior to the conception to carry a baby to term for a couple.

Testicles. The sexual glands in a man where sperm are produced.

Ultrasound. Also called pulse-echo sonography; a technique for visualizing the fetus in the uterus that allows for estimating the size and detecting some abnormalities.

Ultrasound-Guided Aspiration. A nonsurgical method for egg retrieval.

Uterus. Womb; the female organ in which the fetus grows during pregnancy.

Varicocele. A varicose vein in the scrotum; may cause infertility.

Vasectomy. Surgery to sterilize a man.

Resources and Organizations

Infertility Organizations and Support Groups

RESOLVE
5 Water Street
Arlington, MA 02174
617/643-2424

This organization is the best resource for information on all aspects of infertility. It is a national member-supported organization for infertile people with local chapters throughout the country. The national office provides links between people who have similar problems, up-to-date bibliographies, lists of specialists, a bimonthly newsletter with current information on treatments and resources, fact sheets on various topics, and telephone counseling.

American Fertility Society
2131 Magnolia Avenue
Birmingham, AL 35256

Professional organization for clinicians and researchers specializing in fertility and publisher of the medical journal *Fertility and Sterility*.

American College of Obstetricians and Gynecologists
600 Maryland Avenue, S.W.
Suite 300 East
Washington, DC 20024

Professional organization of board-certified obstetricians and gynecologists. It can provide a list of specialists in your area.

The following are self-help organizations that provide information and support. They offer educational resources, networking, and information about local chapters.

Endometriosis Association
P.O. Box 92187
Milwaukee, WI 53202

Turner's Syndrome Support Group of New England
% Drusilla Davis
170 Maple Street
Malden, MA 02148
617/322-4792

DES Action National Offices
Long Island Jewish Hillside Medical Center
New Hyde Park, NY 11040

HERS: Hysterectomy Educational Resources and Services
501 Woodbrook Lane
Philadelphia, PA 19119

Pregnancy Loss Support

SHARE
% Sister Jane Marie Lamb
St. John's Hospital
800 E. Carpenter St.
Springfield, IL 62702
217/544-6464, ext. 4500

A national network of over three hundred local support groups for families that have experienced miscarriage, ectopic pregnancy, stillbirth, or infant death. The national office publishes a newsletter and provides resource material for families and for support groups.

The Compassionate Friends, Inc.
P.O. Box 1347
Oak Brook, IL 60521
313/323-5010

A self-help organization for parents whose children have died at any age or who have suffered a pregnancy loss. Chapters exist throughout the world.

Loving Arms (Pregnancy and Infant Loss Center)
1415 E. Wayzata Boulevard
Suite 22
Wayzata, MN 55391

An organization providing resources and educational materials on pregnancy loss.

Adoption Resources

OURS, Inc. (Organization for United Response)
207 Highway 100 North
Suite 203
Minneapolis, MN 55422

A national network of support groups concerned with the adoption of foreign-born children. It provides information and support for both adoptive and prospective adoptive families. It has over one hundred local chapters in the United States.

National Committee for Adoption (NCFA)
1346 Connecticut Avenue, N.W.
Suite 326
Washington, DC 20036

A resource and lobbying organization that provides information about adoption agencies, adoption practices, and the impact of current adoption methods.

Parents for Private Adoption
P.O. Box 7
Pawlet, VT 05761

**North American Council on Adoptable Children
(NACAC)**
810 18th Street, N.W.
Suite 703
Washington, DC 20006

An organization that publishes *Adoptalk* and provides information about adoption and local parent groups in the United States
and Canada.

Women's Organizations

Groups that are examining the impact of reproductive technology on women include:

Boston Women's Health Book Collective
47 Nicholes Avenue
Watertown, MA 02172

FINRRAGE
**(Feminist International Network Resisting Reproductive
and Genetic Engineering)**
P.O. Box 441216
West Somerville, MA 02144

Fertility Programs

There are thousands of fertility programs in North America. Because of the growing demand, new centers are opening all the
time. However, some, particularly IVF and surrogate programs,
do not last very long. Therefore, rather than publish a list that
will be quickly outdated, we are providing addresses of organizations from which the most current information can be obtained.

Having the name of a nearby clinic or specialist is not sufficient. Make sure a physician who calls him or herself a specialist
actually has extra training and preferably is board certified to
treat infertility. Ask fertility centers about their costs and about
the range of medical and psychological services they provide. Be

sure you know their actual track record, not just their claims or the national averages. If you're not satisfied with the answers, keep looking—there may be a better program a little farther away.

Artificial Insemination

The American Fertility Society, the American College of Obstetricians and Gynecologists, and RESOLVE all maintain lists of fertility specialists who do artificial insemination (see addresses in earlier section).

In Vitro Fertilization

The American Fertility Society has the most complete list of IVF programs. In addition, RESOLVE has a list of all of the clinics that responded to a questionnaire. This list includes more complete information obtained from the questionnaire about each program. (See address in earlier section.)

Surrogate Motherhood

RESOLVE maintains the most up-to-date list of programs. (See address in earlier section.)

Ovum Transfer

Fertility and Genetics Research is the company that is establishing OT centers. It can be reached for further information at 624 South Grand Avenue, Suite 2900, Los Angeles, CA 90017.

Notes

Introduction

1. Susan Borg and Judith Lasker, *When Pregnancy Fails: Families Coping with Miscarriage, Stillbirth, and Infant Death* (Boston: Beacon Press, 1981).

2. Merle J. Berger and Donald P. Goldstein, "Infertility Related to Exposure to DES *in utero:* Reproductive Problems in the Female," in Miriam D. Mazor and Harriet F. Simons, eds., *Infertility: Medical Emotional, and Social Considerations* (New York: Human Sciences Press, 1984), 157–68 ◆Daniel Cramer et al., "Tubal Infertility and the Intrauterine Device," *New England Journal of Medicine,* 312 (1985), 941 ◆Elina Hemminki, B. I. Graubard, H. J. Hoffman, W. D. Mosher, and K. Fetterly, "Cesarean Section and Subsequent Fertility: Results from the 1982 National Survey of Family Growth," *Fertility and Sterility* 43 (April 1985): 520–28 ◆Gerry Hendershot, "Maternal Age and Overdue Conceptions," *American Journal of Public Health* 74 (January 1984): 35–37 ◆Jane Menken, J. Trussel, and U. Larsen, "Age and Infertility," *Science,* September 26, 1986, 1389–94. ◆William D. Mosher and Sevgi O. Aral, "Factors Related to Infertility in the United States, 1965–1976," *Sexually Transmitted Diseases,* July–September 1985, 117–23 ◆Alan B. Retik and Stuart B. Bauer, "Infertility Related to DES Exposure *in utero:* Reproductive Problems in the Male," in Mazor and Simons, *Infertility,* 169–79.

3. In addition, an estimated 9.5 million women are in couples in which one partner was sterilized for contraceptive purposes. Yet one-fourth of these women express the desire for a future pregnancy and may be candidates for one of the methods described here. The image

presented in the media of infertility being a problem increasingly affecting mostly professional women in their thirties is misleading. Infertility rates have actually risen in only one age-group—women between twenty and twenty-four years of age. Infertility is also twice as likely to affect black women as white women, and most black women are not in the upper middle class, which has received so much attention. William Mosher, "Reproductive Impairments in the United States, 1965–1982," *Demography* 22 (August 1985): 415–29; Sevgi O. Aral and William Cates, "The Increasing Concern with Infertility—Why Now?" *Journal of the American Medical Association,* November 4, 1983, 2327–31; Mosher and Aral, "Factors Related to Infertility in the United States."

4. A sampling of recent important works: ◆Lori Andrews, *New Conceptions: A Consumer's Guide to the Newest Infertility Treatments* (New York: Ballantine, 1985) ◆Rita Arditti, Renata Duelli Klein, and Shelly Minden, eds., *Test Tube Women: What Future for Motherhood?* (Boston: Pandora Press, 1984) ◆Gena Corea, *The Mother Machine: Reproductive Technologies from Artificial Insemination to Artificial Wombs* (New York: Harper and Row, 1985) ◆Sherman Elias and George Annas, "Social Policy Considerations in Noncoital Reproduction," *Journal of the American Medical Association,* January 3, 1986, 62–68 ◆Helen Holmes, Betty Hoskins, and Michael Gross, eds., *The Custom-Made Child: Women-Centered Perspectives* (Englewood Cliffs, N.J.: Humana Press, 1981) ◆Peter Singer and Deane Wells, *Making Babies: The New Science and Ethics of Conception* (New York: Scribner, 1985) ◆R. Snowden, G. D. Mitchell, and E. M. Snowden, *Artificial Reproduction: A Social Investigation* (London: George Allen and Unwin, 1983).

5. "When Baby's Mother is Also Grandma—and Sister," Case Studies, *Hastings Center Report* 15 (1985): 29–31 ◆Barbara Katz Rothman, "How Science Is Redefining Parenthood," *Ms.,* August 1982, 154–58.

Chapter 1: The Drive to Have Children

1. Lesley Brown and John Brown, with Sue Freeman, *Our Miracle Called Louise: A Parents' Story* (New York and London: Paddington Press, 1979).

2. Edward O. Wilson, *Sociobiology: The New Synthesis* (Cambridge: Harvard University Press, 1975) ◆Jessie Bernard, *The Future of Motherhood* (New York: Penguin, 1974) ◆Diana Burgwyn, *Marriage without Children* (New York: Harper and Row, 1981) ◆Betty Friedan, *The Feminine Mystique: Twentieth Anniversary Edition* (New York: Norton, 1983) ◆Ellen Peck and Judith Senderowitz, eds.,

Pronatalism: The Myth of Mom and Apple Pie (New York: Thomas Y. Crowell, 1974) ♦J. Richard Udry, "The Effect of Normative Pressures on Fertility," *Population and Environment: Behavioral and Social Issues* 5 (Summer 1982): 109–22 ♦Jean Veevers, "Voluntary Childlessness: A Review of Issues and Evidence," *Marriage and Family Review* 2 (1979): 1–26.

3. P. H. Jamison, Louis R. Franzini, and Robert M. Kaplan, "Some Assumed Characteristics of Voluntarily Childfree Women and Men," *Psychology of Women Quarterly* 4 (1979): 266–73 ♦Marcia Ory, "The Decision to Parent or Not: Normative and Structural Components," *Journal of Marriage and the Family* 40 (August 1978): 531–39.

4. Charles Westoff, "Fertility in The United States," *Science,* October 31, 1986, 554–59.

5. Judy Klemesrud, "Single Mothers by Choice: Perils and Joys," *New York Times,* May 2, 1983, 35 ♦Maureen McGuire and Nancy Alexander, "Artificial Insemination of Single Women," *Fertility and Sterility* 43 (February 1985): 182–84.

6. Nancy Felipe Russo, "The Motherhood Mandate," *Journal of Social Issues* 32 (1976): 143–53.

7. Norval D. Glenn, "Psychological Well-being in the Post-Parental Stage: Some Evidence from National Surveys," *Journal of Marriage and the Family* 37 (February 1975): 105–10 ♦Norval Glenn and Sara McLanahan, "Children and Marital Happiness: A Further Specification of the Relationship," *Journal of Marriage and the Family* 44 (February 1982): 63–72 ♦Sharon Houseknecht, "Childlessness and Marital Adjustment," *Journal of Marriage and the Family* 41 (May 1979): 259–65 ♦Richard Lerner and Spanier Graham, eds., *Child Influences on Marital and Family Interaction* (New York: Academic Press, 1978).

8. Elaine Hilberman Carmen, N. F. Russo, and J. B. Miller, "Inequality and Women's Mental Health: An Overview," *American Journal of Psychiatry* 138 (October 1981): 1319–30 ♦Walter Gove and M. Hughes, "Possible Causes of the Apparent Sex Difference in Physical Health," *American Sociological Review* 44 (1979): 126–46 ♦Walter Gove and J. F. Tudor, "Adult Sex Roles and Mental Illness," *American Journal of Sociology* 78 (1973): 50–73 ♦Holly Waldron and Donald Routh, "The Effect of the First Child on the Marital Relationship," *Journal of Marriage and the Family* 43 (November 1981): 785–88.

9. Erving Goffman, *Stigma* (Englewood Cliffs, N.J.: Prentice Hall, 1963) ♦Charlene Miall, "The Stigma of Involuntary Childlessness," *Social Problems* 33 (1986): 268–82 ♦Jean Veevers, "The Violation of Fertility Mores: Voluntary Childlessness as Deviant Behavior," in Craig Boydell, Craig F. Grindstaff, and Paul C. Whitehead, eds., *Deviant Behavior and Societal Reaction* (New York: Holt Rinehart and Winston, 1973).

10. Edmond J. Farris and Mortimer Garrison, "Emotional Impact of Successful Donor Insemination," *Obstetrics and Gynecology* 3 (1954): 19–20.

11. Jeannette E. Given, G. S. Jones, and D. L. McMillen, "A Comparison of Personality Characteristics between In Vitro Fertilization Patients and Other Infertile Patients," *Journal of In Vitro Fertilization and Embryo Transfer* 2 (1985): 49–54.

Chapter 2: Feelings of Grief

1. Kathleen McGinnis-Craft, "Once Again," *RESOLVE Newsletter,* September 1985, 5.

2. Jill Woodcliff, "Changing," *RESOLVE Newsletter,* April 1985, 8.

3. Erich Lindemann, "Symptomatology and Management of Acute Grief," *American Journal of Psychiatry* 101 (1944): 141–48 ◆Anne Martin Matthews and Ralph Matthews, "Beyond the Mechanics of Infertility: Perspectives on the Social Psychology of Infertility and Involuntary Childlessness," *Family Relations* 35 (October 1986): 479–87 ◆Barbara Eck Menning, "The Emotional Needs of Infertile Couples," *Fertility and Sterility* 34 (October 1980): 313–19.

4. Patricia Mahlstedt, "The Psychological Component of Infertility," *Fertility and Sterility* 43 (March 1985): 341.

5. Janet Daling et al., "Tubal Infertility in Relation to Prior Induced Abortion," *Fertility and Sterility* 43 (March 1985): 389–94.

6. Miriam Mazor, "Emotional Reactions to Infertility," in *Infertility: Medical Emotional and Social Considerations* (New York: Human Science Press, 1984), 23–35 ◆Helene Deutsch, *The Psychology of Women* (New York: Grune and Stratton, 1945) ◆F. M. Mai, "The Diagnosis and Treatment of Psychogenic Infertility," *Infertility* 1 (1978): 109 ◆Matthews and Matthews, "Mechanics of Infertility" ◆Philip Sarrel and Alan H. DeCherney, "Psychotherapeutic Intervention for Treatment of Couples with Secondary Infertility," *Fertility and Sterility* 43 (June 1985): 897–900.

7. Mazor, "Emotional Reactions to Infertility."

8. Linda P. Salzer, *Infertility: How Couples Can Cope* (Boston: G. K. Hall, 1986).

9. Gjerde Dausch, "Secondary Infertility: A Personal Experience," *RESOLVE Newsletter,* April 1982, 5.

Other suggested readings: ◆Merle Bombardieri, "Coping with the Stress of Infertility," publication from RESOLVE, 1984 ◆Marie Chevret, "Problems Related to Requests for AID and Psychological Assistance Offered to Couples," in G. David and W. Price, eds., *Human Artificial Insemination and Semen Preservation* (New York: Plenum

Press, 1980) ♦Dorothy Greenfield, C. Mazure, F. Haseltine, and A. De-Cherney, "The Role of the Social Worker in the In-Vitro Fertilization Program," *Social Work in Health Care* 10 (Winter 1984): 49–54 ♦Barbara Eck Menning, *Infertility: A Guide for the Childless Couple* (Englewood Cliffs, N.J.: Prentice-Hall, 1977) ♦Wulf Utian, James Goldfarb, and Miriam Rosenthal, "Psychological Aspects of Infertility," in L. Dennerstein and G. D. Burrows, eds., *Handbook of Psychosomatic Obstetrics and Gynaecology* (New York: Elsevier Biomedical, 1983) ♦Anne Woollett, "Childlessness: Strategies for Coping with Infertility," *International Journal of Behavioral Development* 8 (1985): 473–82 ♦William J. Worden, *Grief Counseling and Grief Therapy: A Handbook for the Mental Health Practitioner* (New York, Springer, 1982).

Chapter 3: Artificial Insemination

1. In 1979, George Annas estimated that 250,000 Americans had been conceived by AID; other experts estimate that an additional 10,000 to 15,000 are being born each year by AID. No estimates exist for babies born from AIH. Therefore 350,000 is probably a conservative number. ♦George J. Annas, "Fathers Anonymous: Beyond the Best Interests of the Sperm Donor," in Aubrey Milunsky and G. Annas, *Genetics and the Law II* (New York: Plenum Press, 1979).

2. Lori Andrews, *New Conceptions: A Consumer's Guide to the Newest Infertility Treatments* (New York: Ballantine, 1985) ♦Erik Bostofte, Jørgen Serup, and Heinrich Rebbe, "Has the Fertility of Danish Men Declined through the Years in Terms of Semen Quality?" *International Journal of Fertility* 28 (1983): 91–95 ♦Jane E. Brody, "Sperm Found Especially Vulnerable to Environment," *New York Times,* March 10, 1981 ♦Cynthia Cooke and Susan Dworkin, "It's Time to Take Male Infertility Seriously," *Ms.,* March 1981, 89–91 ♦Katherine Bouton, "Fighting Male Infertility," *New York Times Magazine,* June 13, 1982, 86–91.

3. Stephen Corson and Frances F. Batzer, "Homologous Artificial Insemination," *Journal of Reproductive Medicine* 26 (May 1981): 909–15 ♦Michael Diamond, G. Lavy, and A. H. DeCherney, "Pregnancy Following Use of the Cervical Cup for Home Artificial Insemination Utilizing Homolegous Semen," *Fertility and Sterility* 39 (April 1983): 480–84 ♦Claude Gernignon and Jean-Marie Kunstmann, "AIH for Semen Insufficiency: 119 Cases," in G. David and W. Price, eds., *Human Artificial Insemination and Semen Preservation* (New York: Plenum Press, 1980) ♦M. Usherwood, "AIH for Cases of Spermatozoa Antibod-

ies and Oligo-zoospermia, in David and Price, *Human Artificial Insemination.*

4. Ethics Committee of the American Fertility Society, "Ethical Considerations of the New Reproductive Technologies," *Fertility and Sterility Supplement* 46 (September 1986): 15–925 ◆Jonathan Hewitt, "Treatment of Idiopathic Infertility, Cervical Mucus Hostility, and Male Infertility: Artificial Insemination with Husband's Semen or In-Vitro Fertilization," *Fertility and Sterility* 44 (September 1985): 350–55 ◆Kamran Moghissi et al., "Homologous Artificial Insemination: A Reappraisal," *American Journal of Obstetrics and Gynecology,* December 15, 1977, 231–42.

5. Nancy Allen et al., "Intrauterine Insemination: A Critical Review," *Fertility and Sterility* 44 (November 1985): 569–80 ◆Roger Toffle et al., "Intrauterine Insemination: The University of Minnesota Experience," *Fertility and Sterility* 43 (May 1985): 743–47.

6. Diane Clapp, "Artificial Insemination by Husband or Donor Sperm," publication of RESOLVE, n.d. ◆Martin Curie-Cohen, L. Luttrell, and S. Shapiro, "Current Practice of Artificial Insemination by Donor in the United States," *New England Journal of Medicine,* March 15, 1979, 585–90.

7. David Berger, "Couples' Reactions to Male Infertility and Donor Insemination" *American Journal of Psychiatry* 137 (September 1980): 1047–49 ◆Laurence Karp, "Artificial Insemination: A Need for Caution," *American Journal of Medical Genetics* 9 (1981): 179–81 ◆W. Thompson and D. D. Boyle, "Counselling Patients for Artificial Insemination and Subsequent Pregnancy," *Clinics in Obstetrics and Gynaecology* 9 (April 1982): 211–25.

8. "More Childless Wives Conceive through Use of Frozen Sperm," *New York Times,* January 8, 1979, 19 ◆Jon H. Alfredsson, S. P. Gudmundsson, and G. Snaedal, "Artificial Insemination by Donor with Frozen Sperm," *Obstetrical and Gynecological Survey* 38 (1983): 305–12.

9. Alfredsson, Gudmundsson, and Snaedal, "Artificial Insemination with Frozen Sperm" ◆Clapp, "Artificial Insemination" ◆G. L. Foss, "Artificial Insemination by Donor: A Review of 12 Years' Experience," *Journal of Biosocial Science* 14 (1982): 253–62 ◆Michael Richter, Ray Haning, and Sanders Shapiro, "AID, Fresh vs Frozen," abstract, *Fertility and Sterility* 39 (March 1983): 397.

10. Andrews, *New Conceptions,* 172.

11. Bernard Rubin, "Psychological Aspects of Human Artificial Insemination," *Archives of General Psychiatry* 13 (August 1965): 121–32.

12. Annas, "Fathers Anonymous."

13. Curie-Cohen, Luttrell, and Shapiro, "Current Practice of Artificial Insemination."

14. "Barn Genom Insemination," (Children through Insemination) *Sou* 42 (1983): 201–19 (English summary).

15. Andrews, *New Conceptions.*

16. Carol Berquist et al., "Artificial Insemination with Fresh Donor Semen Using the Cervical Cap Technique: A Review of 278 Cases," *Obstetrics and Gynecology* 60 (August 1982): 195–99.

17. Ibid.; G. L. Foss, "Artificial Insemination by Donor" ♦Stephen Corson, F. R. Batzer, and M. M. Baylson, "Donor Insemination," *Obstetrics and Gynecology Annual* 12 (1983): 283–309 ♦Curie-Cohen, Luttrell, and Shapiro, "Current Practice of Artificial Insemination."

18. Rubin, "Psychological Aspects."

19. Alan F. Guttmacher, "The Role of Artificial Insemination in the Treatment of Sterility," *Obstetric and Gynecologic Survey* 15 (1960): 761–85.

20. B. I. Somfai and A. Lynch, "A Judeo-Christian Evaluation of Artificial Insemination and Its Implication to Embryo Transfer," *Archives of Andrology* 5 (1980): 50.

21. R. Snowden, G. D. Mitchell, and E. M. Snowden, *Artificial Reproduction: A Social Investigation* (London: George Allen and Unwin, 1983).

22. J. C. Czyba and M. Chevret, "Psychological Reactions of Couples to Artificial Insemination with Donor Sperm," *International Journal of Fertility* 24 (1979): 240–45 ♦R. S. Ledward, E. M. Symonds, and S. Eynon, "Social and Environmental Factors as Criteria for Success in Artificial Insemination by Donor," *Journal of Biosocial Science* 14 (1982): 263–75.

23. Aphrodite Clamar, "Psychological Implications of Donor Insemination," *American Journal of Psychoanalysis* 40 (1980): 176.

24. Gena Corea, *The Mother Machine: Reproductive Technologies from Artificial Insemination to Artificial Wombs* (New York: Harper and Row, 1985) ♦Maureen McGuire and Nancy Alexander, "Artificial Insemination of Single Women," *Fertility and Sterility* 43 (February 1985): 182–84 ♦Carson Strong and Jay Schinfeld, "The Single Woman and Artificial Insemination by Donor," *Journal of Reproductive Medicine* 29 (May 1984): 293–99.

25. Curie-Cohen, Luttrell, and Shapiro, "Current Practice of Artificial Insemination."

26. Ian Milsom and Per Bergman, "A Study of Parental Attitudes after Donor Insemination," *Acta Obstetrica et Gynecologica Scandinavica* (1982): 125–28 ♦Sue Teper and E. Malcolm Symonds, "Artificial Insemination by Donor: Problems and Perspectives," in Cedric Carter, ed., *Developments in Human Reproduction and Their Eugenic and Ethical Implications* (London: Academic Press, 1982).

Other suggested references: ♦S. J. Behrman, "Artificial Insemination," *Clinical Obstetrics and Gynecology* 22 (March 1979):

245–53 ◆Kenneth Borg, "A Legal Overview of Artificial Insemina-tion," typescript ◆Karen Gruber D'Andrea, "The Role of the Nurse Practitioner in Artificial Insemination," *Journal of Obstetric, Gyneco-logic, and Neonatal Nursing* 13 (March/April 1984): 75–78 ◆Brent J. Jensen, "Artificial Insemination and the Law," *Brigham Young Univer-sity Law Review,* 1982, 935 ◆John Leeton and June Backwell, "A Pre-liminary Psychosocial Follow-Up of Parents and Their Children Con-ceived by Artificial Insemination by Donor," *Clinical Reproduction and Fertility* 1 (1982): 307–10 ◆Malkah Notman, "Psychological Aspects of AID," in Miriam D. Mazor and Harriet Simons, eds., *Infertility: Med-ical, Emotional, and Social Considerations* (New York: Human Sci-ence Press, 1984), 145–53 ◆Anthony Reading, C. M. Sledmere, and D. N. Cox, "A Survey of Patient Attitudes towards Artificial Insemination by Donor," *Journal of Psychosomatic Research* 26 (1982): 429–33 ◆R. Snowden and G. D. Mitchell, *The Artificial Family: A Consideration of Artificial Insemination by Donor* (London: George Allen and Unwin, 1981) ◆W. Thompson and D. D. Boyle, "Counselling Patients for Artificial Insemination and Subsequent Pregnancy," *Clinics in Obstetrics and Gynaecology* 9 (April 1982): 211–25 ◆John P. P. Tyler, M. K. Nicholas, N. G. Crockett, and G. L. Driscoll, "Some Attitudes to Artificial Insemination by Donor," *Clinical Reproduction and Fer-tility* 2 (1983): 151–60.

Chapter 4: In Vitro Fertilization

1. Michael Gold, "The Baby Makers," *Science* 85 (April 1985): 26–38 ◆Howard Jones, "In Vitro Fertilization: Past, Present, and Fu-ture," presentation at Lehigh University, October 14, 1986.

2. C. Campagnoli, A. DiGregorio, R. Arisio, and L. Fessia, "Patient Selection for In Vitro Fertilization and Embryo Transfer," *Experientia,* December 15, 1985, 1491–93 ◆Claudio Chillik, "The Role of In Vitro Fertilization in Infertile Patients with Endometriosis," *Fertility and Ste-rility* 44 (July 1985): 56–61 ◆Jacques Cohen et al., "In Vitro Fertil-ization: A Treatment for Male Infertility," *Fertility and Sterility* 43 (March 1985): 422–32 ◆Patrick Steptoe, "The Selection of Couples for In Vitro Fertilization and Embryo Replacement," *Annals New York Academy of Sciences* 442 (1985): 487–89.

3. Gold, "Baby Makers."

4. Jacques Cohen et al., "In Vitro Fertilization Using Cryopreserved Donor Semen in Cases Where Both Partners Are Infertile," *Fertility and Sterility* 43 (April 1985): 570–74 ◆Maha Mahadeven, A. D. Trounson, and J. F. Leeton, "Successful Use of Human Semen Cryobanking for In Vitro Fertilization," *Fertility and Sterility* 40 (September 1983):

340–43 ♦Alan Trounson, J. Leeton, M. Besanko, C. Wood, and A. Conti, "Pregnancy Established in an Infertile Patient after Transfer of a Donated Embryo Fertilized In Vitro," *British Medical Journal* 286 (March 1983): 835–38.

5. Gina Kolata, "Ethical Guidelines Proposed for Reproductive Technology," *Science,* September 9, 1986, 1255 ♦Michael R. Soules, "The In Vitro Fertilization Pregnancy Rate: Let's Be Honest with One Another," *Fertility and Sterility* 43 (April 1985): 511–13.

6. J. Dor, "Successful In Vitro Fertilization and Embryo Transfer in a Group of Patients with Tubal Infertility," *Israel Journal of Medical Sciences* 20 (1984): 41–45 ♦Howard H. Jones et al., "What Is a Pregnancy? A Question for Programs of In Vitro Fertilization," *Fertility and Sterility* 40 (December 1983): 728–33 ♦Maha Mahadevan, "The Relationship of Tubal Blockage, Infertility of Unknown Cause, Suspected Male Infertility, and Endometrosis to Success of In Vitro Fertilization and Embryo Transfer," *Fertility and Sterility* 40 (December 1983): 755–62 ♦Robert Visscher, H. A. Moore, and M. Hager, "In Vitro Fertilization in a Community Hospital," *Fertility and Sterility* 44 (December 1985): 822–26.

7. Georgeanna Jones, "Update on In Vitro Fertilization," *Endocrine Reviews* 5 (1984): 62–75.

8. Diane Clapp, "Medical Updates: G.I.F.T.," *RESOLVE Newsletter,* June 1985, 6 ♦Jon Van, " 'Test Tube Baby' Technique Matures," *Morning Call,* Allentown, Pa., March 25, 1986, D4.

9. Alan Trounson, "Current Perspectives of In Vitro Fertilization and Embryo Transfer," *Clinical Reproduction and Fertility* 1 (1982): 55–65 ♦Personal communication, 1987.

10. Ellen Freeman, A. S. Boxer, K. Rickels, R. Tureck, and L. Mastroianni, Jr., "Psychological Evaluation and Support in Program of In Vitro Fertilization and Embryo Transfer, *Fertility and Sterility* 43 (January 1985): 48–53 ♦F. P. Haseltine et al., "Psychological Interviews in Screening Couples Undergoing In Vitro Fertilization," *Annals New York Academy of Sciences* 442 (1985): 504–22.

11. Ken Mao and Carl Wood, "Barriers to Treatment of Infertility by In Vitro Fertilization and Embryo Transfer," *Medical Journal of Australia* 140 (April 1984): 532–33.

12. Australian In Vitro Collaborative Group, "High Incidence of Preterm Births and Early Losses in Pregnancy after In Vitro Fertilization, *British Medical Journal,* October 26, 1985, 1160–63 ♦S. Trotnow, S. Al-Hasani, T. Hunlich, and W. B. Schill, "Bilateral Tubal Pregnancy Following In Vitro Fertilization and Embryo Transfer," *Archives of Gynecology* 234 (1983): 75–78 ♦John Yovich, "Embryo Transfer Technique as a Cause of Ectopic Pregnancies in In Vitro Fertilization," *Fertility and Sterility* 44 (September 1985): 318.

13. A. Demoulin, R. Bologne, J. Hustin, and R. Lambotte, "Is Ultrasound Monitoring of Follicular Growth Harmless?" *Annals of New York Academy of Sciences* 442 (1985): 146–52 ◆Melvin Stratmeyer and Christopher Christman, "Biological Effects of Ultrasound," *Women and Health* 7 (1982): 65–81.

14. Susan Lenz and Jorgen Lauritsen, "Ultrasonically Guided Percutaneous Aspiration of Human Follicles under Local Anesthesia: A New Method of Collecting Oocytes for In Vitro Fertilization," *Fertility and Sterility* 38 (December 1982): 673–77 ◆Matts Wikland, L. Enk, and L. Hamberger, "Transvesical and Transvaginal Approaches for the Aspiration of Follicles by Use of Ultrasound," *Annals of New York Academy of Sciences* 442 (1985): 146–52.

15. John Biggers, "Risks of In Vitro Fertilization and Embryo Transfer in Humans," *In Vitro Fertilization and Embryo Transfer,* 1983, 393 ◆John Henahan, "Fertilization, Embryo Transfer Procedures Raise Many Questions," *Journal of American Medical Association* August 17, 1984, 877–82 ◆James Schlesselman, "How Does One Assess the Risk of Abnormalities from Human In Vitro Fertilization?" *American Journal of Obstetrics and Gynecology,* September 1, 1979, 135–48.

16. John Kerin, "Incidence of Multiple Pregnancy after In Vitro Fertilization and Embryo Transfer," *Lancet,* September 3, 1983, 537–40.

17. Constance Holden, "Two Fertilized Eggs Stir Global Fervor," *Science,* July 6, 1984, 35 ◆Alan Trounson, "In Vitro Fertilization, Problems of the Future," *British Journal of Hospital Medicine* 31 (February 1984): 104–6.

18. Ethics Advisory Board, *Report and Conclusions: HEW Support of Research Involving Human In Vitro Fertilization and Embryo Transfer* (Washington, D.C.: DHEW, 1979) ◆Peter Singer and Diane Wells, "In Vitro Fertilization: The Major Issues," *Journal of Medical Ethics* 9 (1983): 192–95.

Other suggested readings: ◆Randall Blow, "In Vitro Fertilization: New Territory for the Preception Tort," *George Mason University Law Review* 5 (1982): 169–83 ◆Diane Clapp, "In Vitro Fertilization: An Overview," *RESOLVE,* Belmont, Mass. ◆Mark Cohen, "The 'Brave New Baby' and the Law: Fashioning Remedies for the Victims of In Vitro Fertilization," *American Journal of Law and Medicine* 4: 319–36 ◆R. G. Edwards and P. C. Steptoe, "Current Status of In Vitro Fertilization and Implantation of Human Embryos," *Lancet,* December 3, 1983, 1265–69 ◆Catherine Garner, "In Vitro Fertilization and Embryo Transfer," *Journal of Obstetric, Gynecologic, and Neonatal Nursing* 12 (March/April 1983): 75–78 ◆Dorothy Greenfield, "The Role of the Social Worker in the In Vitro Fertilization Program," *Social Work in Health Care* 10 (Winter 1984): 49–54 ◆Clifford Grobstein, M. Flower, and J. Mendeloff, "External Human Fertilization: An Evaluation of Policy," *Science,* October 14, 1983, 127–33 ◆Michael Kramer, "Last Chance Babies," *New York,* August 12, 1985, 34–42 ◆Marc Lappe, "Ethics at the Center of Life: Protecting Vulnerable Subjects," *Hastings Center Report* 8 (October 1978): 11–13 ◆Richard Marrs, "A Modified Technique of Human In Vitro Fertilization and Embryo Transfer," *American Journal of Obstetrics and Gynecology,* October 1, 1983, 318–22 ◆Hugh Melnick, "Clinical Aspects of In Vitro Fertilization," *Female Patient* 9 (October 1984): 115–23 ◆Pat Ohlerdorf, "Beyond the Limits of Life," *Maclean's,* November 15, 1982, 52–59 ◆Paul Ramsey, "Manufacturing Our Offspring: Weighing the Risks," *Hastings Center Report* 8 (October 1978): 79 ◆John Robertson, "In Vitro Conception and Harm to the Unborn," *Hastings Center Report* 8 (October 1978): 13–17 ◆Geoffrey Sher, "The Development of a Successful Non-University Based Ambulatory In Vitro Fertilization/Embryo Transfer Program: Phase 1," *Fertility and Sterility,* April 1984, 511–17 ◆Melvin Taymor, "Current Status of In Vitro Fertilization and Reimplantation," in Aubrey Milunsky and George Annas, eds., *Genetics and the Law II* (New York: Plenum Press, 1979), 345–50 ◆Stephen Toulmin, "In Vitro Fertilization: Answering the Ethical Objectives," *Hastings Center Report* 8 (October 1978): 9–11 ◆LeRoy Walters, "Human In Vitro Fertilization: A Review of the Ethical Literature," *Hastings Center Report* 9 (August 1979): 23–43 ◆William Walters and Peter Singer, eds., *Test-Tube Babies: A Guide to Moral Questions, Present Techniques and Future Possibilities* (Melbourne, Australia: Oxford University Press, 1984) ◆Charles Wilkes, Z. Rosenwaks, D. L. Jones, and H. W. Jones, Jr., "Pregnancy Related to Infertility Diagnosis, Number of Attempts, and Age in a Program of In Vitro Fertilization," *Obstetrics and Gynecology* 66 (September 1985): 350–52.

Chapter 5: Surrogate Motherhood

1. Cynthia Gorney, "For Love and Money," *California,* October 1983, 91.

2. Gena Corea, *The Mother Machine: Reproductive Technologies from Artificial Insemination to Artificial Wombs* (New York: Harper and Row, 1985) ◆Ethics Committee of the American Fertility Society, "Ethical Considerations of the New Reproductive Technologies," *Fertility and Sterility Supplement* 46 (September 1986): 15–925 ◆John Robertson, "Surrogate Mothers: Not So Novel after All," *Hastings Center Report* 13 (October 1983): 28–34.

3. See text and footnotes to chap. 11.

4. Robertson, "Surrogate Mothers."

5. Noel Keane, with Dennis Breo, *The Surrogate Mother* (New York: Everest House, 1981); Carol Lawson, "Surrogate Mothers Grow in Numbers Despite Questions," *New York Times,* October 1, 1986, C1, C18.

6. Keane and Breo, *Surrogate Mother.*

7. Lawson, "Surrogate Mothers Grow in Number" ◆Joe Starita, "Battle for Baby Making History," *Miami Herald,* September 8, 1986, 1A, 4A ◆Robert Hanley, "Whitehead Outlines Her Life before Baby M," *New York Times,* February 10, 1987, B1, B15 ◆"Contract Enforced in Child's 'Best Interests' " (Baby M decision by Judge Harvey R. Sorkow), 119 *New Jersey Law Journal* (April 16, 1987): 29–41.

8. Annette Alve, "Surrogate Mothering: What's the Law?" *Redbook,* May 1984, 46 ◆Angela Holder, "Surrogate Motherhood: Babies for Fun and Profit," *Law, Medicine, and Health Care* 12 (June 1984): 115–17 ◆Cynthia Rushevsky, "Legal Recognition of Surrogate Gestation," *Women's Rights Law Reporter* 7 (Winter 1982): 107–42.

Other suggested readings: ◆George Annas, "Contracts to Bear a Child: Compassion or Commercialism?" *Hastings Center Report* 11 (April 1981): 23–24 ◆Barbara Cohen, "Surrogate Mothers: Whose Baby Is It?" *American Journal of Law and Medicine* 10 (Fall 1984): 243–85 ◆David Gehman and Daniel Shapiro, "Infertility: Babies by Contract," *Newsweek,* November 4, 1985, 74–77 ◆Steven R. Gersz, "The Contract in Surrogate Motherhood: A Review of the Issues," *Law, Medicine and Health Care* 12 (June 1984): 107–14 ◆Marilyn Johnston as told to Sara Nelson, "I Gave Birth to Another Woman's Baby," *Redbook,* May 1984, 45–46 ◆Philip J. Parker, "The Psychology of the Pregnant Surrogate Mother: A Newly Updated Report of a Longitudinal Pilot Study," paper presented at American Orthopsychiatric Association meeting, Toronto, April 1984 ◆idem, "Surrogate Motherhood, Psychiatric Screening and Informed Consent, Baby Selling, and Public Policy," *Bulletin of American Academy of Psychiatry and Law* 12 (1984): 21–39 ◆idem, "Surrogate Motherhood: The Interaction of Litigation, Legislation, and Psychiatry," *International Journal of Law and Psychiatry* 5 (1983): 341–54.

Chapter 6: Ovum Transfer

1. "Breeding Bonanza: Embryo Swaps Yield Cows Many Calves Each Year," *Wall Street Journal,* May 9, 1979, 1, 39.

2. Fern Chapman, "Going for Gold in the Baby Business," *Fortune,* September 17, 1984, 41–77 ◆Hal Lancaster, "Firm Offering Human-Embryo Transfers for Profit Stirs Legal and Ethical Debates," *Wall Street Journal,* March 7, 1984, 33 ◆Martin Stuart-Harle, "Making a Buck on Babies," *Globe and Mail,* Toronto, April 19, 1984, L1.

3. Information about possible reasons for using OT and about the research on OT is derived from the following sources: ♦Harris Brotman, "Human Embryo Transplants," *New York Times Magazine,* January 8, 1984 ♦John E. Buster and Mark V. Sauer, "Nonsurgical Donor Ovum Transfer: New Option for Infertile Couples," *Contemporary OB/GYN,* August 1986, 39–48 ♦John E. Buster, Maria Bustillo, et al., "Biologic and Morphologic Development of Donated Human Ova Recovered by Nonsurgical Uterine Lavage," *American Journal of Obstetrics and Gynecology,* September 15, 1985, 211–17 ♦Maria Bustillo, John E. Buster, et al., "Nonsurgical Ovum Transfer as a Treatment in Infertile Women," *Journal of the American Medical Association,* March 2, 1984, 1171–73 ♦FGR Information Packet, Fertility and Genetics Research, Inc., Los Angeles, Calif.

4. Anne Marie C. Kelly, "Psychological Interviews with Ovum Transfer Candidates," paper presented at the American Psychological Association meetings, Anaheim, Calif., 1983.

5. Buster and Sauer, "Nonsurgical Donor Ovum Transfer: New Option for Infertile Couples" ♦Buster et al., "Biologic and Morphologic Development of Donated Human Ova Recovered by Nonsurgical Uterine Lavage" ♦Bustillo et al., "Nonsurgical Ovum Transfer as a Treatment in Infertile Women."

6. Brotman, "Human Embryo Transplants" ♦Buster and Sauer, "Nonsurgical Donor Ovum Transfer" ♦Buster et al., "Biologic and Morphologic Development of Donated Human Ova Recovered by Nonsurgical Uterine Lavage" ♦Bustillo et al., "Nonsurgical Ovum Transfer as a Treatment in Infertile Women" ♦FGR Information Packet.

7. Ethics Committee of the American Fertility Society, "Ethical Considerations of the New Reproductive Technologies," *Fertility and Sterility Supplement* 46 (September 1986): 15–92.

8. John Jenkins, "Fertility Rights," *TWA Ambassador,* January 1985, 60–62.

9. Stuart-Harle, "Making a Buck on Babies."

10. George J. Annas, "Surrogate Embryo Transfer: The Perils of Patenting," *Hastings Center Report,* June 1984, 25–26 ♦Brotman, "Human Embryo Transplants."

11. Stuart-Harle, "Making a Buck on Babies."

Other suggested readings: ♦Grace Ganz Blumberg, "Legal Issues in Nonsurgical Human Ovum Transfer," *Journal of the American Medical Association,* March 2, 1984, 1178–81 ♦Transcript #08223, "Donahue Show," Multimedia Entertainment, Inc., Syndication Services, Cincinnati, Ohio ♦David J. Martin, "MMPI Profiles of Ovum Transfer Donors and Recipients," paper presented at the American Psychological Association meetings, Anaheim, Calif., 1983 ♦LeRoy Walters, "Ethical

Aspects of Surrogate Embryo Transfer," *Journal of the American Medical Association,* October 28, 1983, 2183–84.

Chapter 7: Donors and Surrogate Mothers

1. D. Franks, "Psychiatric Evaluation of Women in a Surrogate Mother Program," *American Journal of Psychiatry* 138 (1981): 1378–79 ♦Hilary Hanafin, "The Surrogate Mother: An Exploratory Study," Ph.D. diss., California School of Professional Psychology, Los Angeles, 1984 ♦Philip J. Parker, "Motivation of Surrogate Mothers: Initial Findings," *American Journal of Psychiatry* 140 (January 1983): 117–18.

2. David J. Handelman, S. M. Dunn, A. J. Conway, L. M. Boylan, and R. P. Jansen, "Psychological and Attitudinal Profiles in Donors for Artificial Insemination," *Fertility and Sterility* 43 (January 1985): 95–101 ♦Patrick Huerre, "Psychological Aspects of Sperm Donation," in G. David and W. S. Price, eds., *Human Artificial Insemination and Semen Preservation* (New York: Plenum Press, 1980), 461–65 ♦Gabor T. Kovacs, C. E. Clayton, and P. McGowan, "The Attitudes of Semen Donors," *Clinical Reproduction and Fertility* 2 (1983): 73–75 ♦Piet Nijs, O. Steeno, and A. Steppe, "Evaluation of AID Donors: Medical and Psychological Aspects," in David and Price, *Human Artificial Insemination,* 453–59. ♦Robyn Rowland, "The Social and Psychological Consequences of Secrecy in Artificial Insemination by Donor (AID) Programmes," *Social Science and Medicine* 21 (1985): 391–96.

3. Martin Curie-Cohen, L. Luttrell, and S. Shapiro, "Current Practice of Artificial Insemination by Donor in the United States," *New England Journal of Medicine,* March 15, 1979, 385–90.

4. Huerre, "Psychological Aspects" ♦Kovacs, Clayton, and McGowan, "Attitudes of Semen Donors."

5. Robyn Rowland, "Attitudes and Opinions of Donors on an Artificial Insemination by Donor (AID) Programme," typescript, Deakin University, Victoria, Australia.

6. Nancy Reame, "Stress and Obstetrical Complications of Pregnancy, Labor, and Delivery with Emphasis on a Surrogate Mother Population," paper presented at American Orthopsychiatric Association, Toronto, April, 1984.

7. Nijs, Steeno, and Steppe, "Evaluation of AIDS Donors."

8. Sandra R. Leiblum and Christopher Barbrack, "AID: A Survey of Attitudes and Knowledge in Medical Students and Infertile Couples," *Journal of Biosocial Science* 15 (1983): 165–72.

9. Gena Corea, *The Mother Machine: Reproductive Technologies from Artificial Insemination to Artificial Wombs* (New York: Harper

and Row, 1985) ◆Ann Snitow, "The Paradox of Birth Technology: Exploring the Good, the Bad, and the Scary," *Ms.*, December 1986, 42–46, 76–77.

10. Philip J. Parker, "The Psychology of the Pregnant Surrogate Mother: A Newly Updated Report of a Longitudinal Pilot Study," paper presented at American Orthopsychiatric Association, Toronto, April 1984.

11. Rowland, "Attitudes and Opinions of Donors."

12. George Annas, "Fathers Anonymous: Beyond the Best Interest of the Sperm Donor," *Family Law Quarterly* 14 (1980): 1–13.

13. Richard Titmuss, *The Gift Relationship* (London: Allen and Unwin, 1971).

Other suggested readings: ◆Paul Bagne, "High-Tech Breeding," *Mother Jones*, August 1983, 23–29, 35 ◆Eva Y. Deykin, L. Campbell, and P. Patti, "The Postadoption Experience of Surrendering Parents," *American Journal of Orthopsychiatry* 54 (1984): 271–80 ◆Anne Taylor Fleming, "New Frontiers in Conception," *New York Times Magazine*, July 20, 1980, 20–24, 42, 48 ◆Karen Mills, "I Had My Sister's Baby," *Ladies' Home Journal*, October 1985, 20–22, 190 ◆Deborah Snyder, as told to John Grossman, "I Was a Surrogate Mother," *Miami Herald*, June 10, 1985.

Chapter 8: The Professionals

1. Alan H. DeCherney, "Doctored Babies," *Fertility and Sterility* 40 (December 1983): 724–27.

2. C. R. Stewart, K. R. Daniels, and J. D. H. Boulnois, "The Development of a Psychosocial Approach to Artificial Insemination of Donor Sperm," *New Zealand Medical Journal*, December 8, 1982, 853–55.

3. F. P. Haseltine et al., "Psychological Interviews in Screening Couples Undergoing In Vitro Fertilization," *Annals of New York Academy of Sciences* 442 (1985): 504–22 ◆W. I. H. Johnston et al., "Patient Selection for In Vitro Fertilization: Physical and Psychological Aspects," *Annals of New York Academy of Sciences* 442 (1985): 490–503.

4. Marcia Millman, *The Unkindest Cut: Life in the Backrooms of Medicine* (New York: Morrow, 1977).

5. Howard Jones, "In Vitro Fertilization: Past, Present, and Future," presentation at Lehigh University, October 14, 1986.

6. Merle A. Bombardieri and Diane Clapp, "Easing Stress for IVF Patients and Staff," *Contemporary OB/GYN*, October 1984, 91–97.

Other suggested readings: ◆Catherine Garner, "In Vitro Fertilization and Embryo Transfer," *Journal of Obstetric, Gynecologic and Neonatal Nursing* 12 (March/April 1983): 75–78 ◆Diane Harris, "What It

Costs to Fight Infertility," *Money,* December 1984, 201–10 ◆Arthur Hoffman and Mary Krell, "Infertility Support Groups," paper presented at Planned Parenthood of Rochester and Monroe County, October 22, 1980 ◆Andrea Shrednick, "Emotional Support Programs for In Vitro Fertilization," *Fertility and Sterility* 40 (1983): 704 ◆W. Thompson and D. D. Boyle, "Counseling Patients for Artificial Insemination and Subsequent Pregnancy," *Clinics in Obstetrics and Gynecology* 9 (April 1982): 211–25.

Chapter 9: The Couple

1. Judith Lorber, "Gender Politics and In Vitro Fertilization Use," paper presented at the Emergency Conference of the Feminist International Network on the New Reproductive Technologies, Sweden, July 3–8, 1985.

2. Lili Hartman, "Thoughts from the Fertile Partner," *RESOLVE Newsletter,* September 1985, 3.

3. Anonymous, "AID Doubts and Feelings," *RESOLVE Newsletter,* December 1985, 2.

4. Giuseppe d'Elicio, Aldo Campana, and L. Mornaghini, "Psychodynamic Discussions with Couples Requesting AID," in G. David and W. Price, eds., *Human Artificial Insemination and Semen Preservation* (New York: Plenum Press, 1980), 409–10.

5. Adrienne Rich, *Of Woman Born: Motherhood as Experience and Institution* (New York: Norton, 1976); Gena Corea, *The Mother Machine* (New York: Harper and Row, 1985); Barbara Katz Rothman, *Giving Birth: Alternatives in Childbirth* (New York: Penguin, 1984), chap. 4.

6. Betty Friedan, *The Second Stage* (New York: Summit Books, 1982); Phyllis Chesler, *With Child* (New York: Berkley Publishing, 1981).

7. "Requests for Contact," *RESOLVE Newsletter,* December 1985, 7.

8. Wulf Utian, James Goldfarb, and Miriam Rosenthal, "Psychological Aspects of Infertility," in L. Dennerstein and G. D. Burrows, eds., *Handbook of Psychosomatic Obstetrics and Gynaecology* (New York: Elsevier Biomedical, 1983), 234.

9. David Berger, "Couples' Reactions to Male Infertility and Donor Insemination," *American Journal of Psychiatry* 137 (September 1980): 1047–49.

Other suggested readings: ◆Claude Alexandre, "Difficulties Encountered by Infertile Couples Facing AID," in David and Price, *Human Artificial Insemination* ◆S. J. Behrman, "Artificial Insemination," *Clinical Obstetrics and Gynecology* 22 (1979): 245–53 ◆David

Berger, "Psychological Aspects of Donor Insemination," *International Journal of Psychiatry in Medicine* 12 (1982): 49–57 ♦Susan Borg and J. Lasker, *When Pregnancy Fails: Families Coping with Miscarriage, Stillbirth, and Infant Death* (Boston: Beacon Press, 1981) ♦Nadine Brozan, "Infertility: Couples' Reactions," *New York Times,* July 26, 1982, 13 ♦Robert Chester, "Is There a Relationship between Childlessness and Marriage Breakdown?" *Journal of Biosocial Science* 4 (1972): 443–54 ♦David Amnon and Dalia Avidan, "Artificial Insemination Donor: Clinical and Psychologic Aspects," *Fertility and Sterility* 27 (May 1976): 528–32 ♦Colin Gibson, "Childlessness and Marital Instability: A Re-Examination of the Evidence," *Journal of Biosocial Science* 12 (1980): 121–32 ♦Arthur Greil and T. A. Leitko, "Couple Decision-Making Regarding Infertility," paper presented to the Society for the Study of Social Problems, New York, August 1986 ♦Carol Gilligan, *In a Different Voice: Psychological Theory and Women's Development* (Cambridge: Harvard University Press, 1982) ♦William Keye, "Psychosexual Responses to Infertility," *Clinical Obstetrics and Gynecology* 27 (September 1984): 760–66 ♦R. S. Ledward, L. Crawford, and E. M. Symonds, "Social Factors in Patients for Artificial Insemination by Donor," *Journal of Biosocial Science* 11 (1979): 473–79 ♦John Leeton and June Blackwell, "A Preliminary Psychosocial Follow-up of Parents and Their Children Conceived by Artificial Insemination by Donor (AID)," *Clinical Reproduction and Fertility* 1 (1982): 307–10 ♦Henri Leridon, "Public Opinion on AID and Sterility," in David and Price, *Human Artificial Insemination* ♦Patricia Mahlstedt, "The Psychological Component of Infertility," *Fertility and Sterility* 43 (March 1985): 335–46 ♦Christine Manuel et al., "Handling of Secrecy by AID Couples," in David and Price, *Human Artificial Insemination* ♦P. Nijs and L. Rouffa, "A.I.D. Couples: Psychological and Psychopathological Evaluation," *Andrologia* 3 (1975): 187–94 ♦Anthony Reading, C. M. Sledmere, and D. N. Cox, "A Survey of Patient Attitudes towards Artificial Insemination by Donor," *Journal of Psychosomatic Research* 26 (1982): 429–33 ♦Hans Rosenkvist, "Donor Insemination," *Danish Medical Bulletin* 28 (September 1981): 133–48 ♦Rosa Salter, "Make a Baby, Break a Marriage," *Morning Call,* Allentown, Pa., May 13, 1986, D-1 ♦Sergio Stone, "Complications and Pitfalls of Artificial Insemination," *Clinical Obstetrics and Gynecology* 23 (September 1980): 667–82 ♦Ronald Strickler, D. W. Keller, and J. C. Warren, "Artificial Insemination with Fresh Donor Semen," *New England Journal of Medicine,* October 23, 1975, 848–53 ♦Herbert Waltzer, "Psychological and Legal Aspects of Artificial Insemination (A.I.D.): An Overview," *American Journal of Psychotherapy* 36 (January 1982): 91–102.

Chapter 10: High-Tech Children

1. James Schlesselman, "How Does One Assess the Risks of Abnormalities from Human In Vitro Fertilization," *American Journal of Obstetrics Gynecology,* September 1979, 135–48 ◆J. F. Mattei and B. LeMarec, "Genetic Aspects of Artificial Insemination by Donor (AID): Indications, Surveillance and Results," *Clinical Genetics* 23 (1983): 132–38.

2. Arthur Sorosky, Annette Baran, and Reuben Pannor, *The Adoption Triangle* (Garden City, N.Y.: Doubleday, 1984).

3. Sorosky, Baran, and Pannor, *Adoption Triangle,* 102–3.

4. Betty Jean Lifton, *Lost and Found: The Adoption Experience* (New York: Dial Press, 1979), 23.

5. Jerome Smith and Franklin Miroff, *You're Our Child: A Social Psychological Approach to Adoption* (Lanham, Md.: University Press of America, 1981), 30 ◆Christine Manuel and Jean-Claude Czyba, "Follow-up Study on Children Born through AID," in G. David and W. S. Price, eds., *Human Artificial Insemination and Semen Preservation* (New York: Plenum Press, 1980), 467–73.

6. Sorosky, Baran, and Pannor, *Adoption Triangle,* chap. 8.

7. Joseph Davis and Dirck Brown, "Artificial Insemination by Donor and the Use of Surrogate Mothers," *Western Journal of Medicine* 141 (July 1984): 128.

8. Jill Krementz, *How It Feels to Be Adopted* (New York: Alfred A. Knopf, 1983), 67.

9. Jean Pierce, "Misconceptions about Adoptive Families," *Early Child Development and Care* 13 (1984): 365–76.

10. Krementz, *How It Feels,* 29.

11. Sorosky, Baran, and Pannor, *Adoption Triangle,* 92.

12. Ibid., chaps. 11 and 12.

13. George Annas, "Artificial Insemination: Beyond the Best Interests of the Donor," *Hastings Center Report* 9 (August 1979): 14–43.

14. Sorosky, Baran, and Pannor, *Adoption Triangle,* 157.

15. Carol Amadio and Stuart Deutsch, "Open Adoption: Allowing Adopted Children to 'Stay in Touch' with Blood Relatives," *Journal of Family Law* 22 (1983/84): 59–93 ◆Reuben Pannor and Annette Baran, "Open Adoption as Standard Practice," *Child Welfare* 63 (May–June 1984): 245–50.

16. Krementz, *How It Feels,* 52.

17. Herbert Waltzer, "Psychological and Legal Aspects of Artificial Insemination (A.I.D.): An Overview," *American Journal of Psychotherapy* 36 (January 1982): 91–102.

18. Lifton, *Lost and Found.*

19. P. K. Snowden, G. D. Mitchell, and E. M. Snowden, *Artificial Reproduction: A Social Investigation* (London: George Allen and Urwin, 1983) ◆Lifton, *Lost and Found.*

20. Snowden, Mitchell, and Snowden, *Artificial Reproduction.*

21. Robert Abramovitz, "Psychological Factors for Children with 'Multiple Parentage,' " paper presented at American Society of Law and Medicine, Cambridge, Massachusetts, October 1984.

22. Elaine Bleckman, "Are Children with One Parent at Psychological Risk? A Methodological Review," *Journal of Marriage and the Family,* February 1982, 179–95.

23. S. Golombok, H. Spencer, and M. Rutter, "Children in Lesbian and Single-Parent Households: Psychosexual and Psychiatric Appraisal," *Journal of Child Psychology and Psychiatry* 24 (1983): 551 ◆R. Green, "Sexual Identity of 37 Children Raised by Homosexual or Transsexual Parents," *American Journal of Psychiatry* 135 (1978): 692 ◆Brenda Maddox, "Homosexual Parents," *Psychology Today,* February 1982, 62–69 ◆Margaret Somerville, "Birth Technology, Parenting and 'Deviance,' " *International Journal of Law and Psychiatry* 5 (1982): 123–53.

24. L. H. Levie, "An Inquiry into the Psychological Effects on Parents of Artificial Insemination with Donor Semen," *Eugenics Review* 59 (1967): 103.

25. John Leeton and June Backwell, "A Preliminary Psychosocial Follow-up of Parents and Their Children Conceived by Artificial Insemination by Donor," *Clinical Reproduction and Fertility* 1 (1982): 307–10 ◆Ian Milsom and Per Bergman, "A Study of Parental Attitudes after Donor Insemination," *Acta Obstetrica et Gynecologica Scandinavica* 16 (1982): 125–28.

26. Krementz, *How It Feels,* 37.

27. Lillian Atallah, "Report from a Test-Tube Baby," *New York Times Magazine,* April 18, 1976, 52.

Other suggested readings: ◆Lori Andrews, "Yours, Mine and Theirs," *Psychology Today,* December 1984, 20–29 ◆Sue Aumend and Marjie Barrett, "Searching and Non-Searching Adoptees," *Adoption and Fostering* (1983): 37–42 ◆idem, "Self-concept and Attitudes toward Adoption: A Comparison of Searching and Nonsearching Adult Adoptees," *Child Welfare* 63 (May–June 1984): 251–59 ◆Maria Berger and Jill Hodges, "Some Thoughts on the Question of When to Tell the Child That He Is Adopted," *Journal of Child Psychotherapy* 8 (1982): 67–87 ◆David Brodzinsky, L. M. Singer, and A. M. Braff, "Children's Understanding of Adoption," *Child Development* 55 (1984): 869–78 ◆J. C. Czyba and M. Chevret, "Psychological Reactions of Couples to Artificial Insemination with Donor Sperm," *International Journal of Fertility* 24 (1979): 240–45 ◆Rita Dukette, "Value Issues in Present-Day Adoption," *Child Welfare* 63 (May–June 1984): 233–43 ◆William Feigelman and Arnold Silverman, *Chosen Children: New Patterns of Adoptive Relationships* (New York: Praeger, 1983) ◆Benson Jaffee and David Fanshel, *How They Fared in Adoption: A Follow-up Study* (New York: Columbia University Press, 1970) ◆Alfred Kadushin, "Adoptive Parenthood: A Hazardous Adventure?" *Social Work* 11 (July 1966): 30–39 ◆Barbara Kritchevsky, "The Unmarried Woman's Right to Artificial Insemination: A Call for an Expanded Definition of Family," *Harvard Women's Law Journal* 4 (1981): 1–4 ◆Maureen McGuire, "Artificial Insemination of Single Women," *Fertility and Sterility* 43 (February 1985): 182–84 ◆Gabriele Semenov, Roger Mises, and Jacqueline Bissery, "Attempt at Follow-up of Children Born through AID," in David and Price, eds., *Human Artificial Insemination,* 475–77 ◆Carson Strong and Jay Schinfeld, "The Single Woman and Artificial Insemination by Donor," *Journal of Reproductive Medicine* 29 (May 1984): 293–99.

Chapter 11: The Reactions of Others

1. "What Do You Think about Test-Tube Babies," *Parents,* November 1978, 148–50.

2. Annette Brodsky, David Martin, Anne Marie Kelly, and Karen Bierman, "Survey of Attitudes about Reproductive Technologies," paper presented at American Psychological Association meetings, Anaheim, Calif., 1983.

3. Robyn Rowland and Coral Ruffin, "Community Attitudes to Artificial Insemination by Husband or Donor, *In Vitro* Fertilization and Adoption," *Clinical Reproduction and Fertility* 21 (1983): 195–206.

4. E. S., "A Womb of One's Own," *Psychology Today,* January 1985, 11.

5. Louis Harris, "The *Life* Poll," *Life Magazine,* June 13, 1969, 52–55.

6. Lori Andrews, *New Conceptions: A Consumer's Guide to the Newest Infertility Treatment* (New York: Ballantine, 1985).

7. "What Do You Think" ◆Glenn M. Vernon and Jack A. Broadway, "Attitudes toward Artificial Insemination and Some Variables Associated Therewith," *Marriage and Family Living* 21 (February 1959): 43–47.

8. Richard L. Matteson and Gerald Terranova, "Social Acceptance of New Techniques of Child Conception," *Journal of Social Psychology* 10 (1977): 225–29.

9. William Tucker, "In Vitro Veritas," *New Republic,* October 28, 1981, 14–16.

10. Theodore Hall, "Test Tube Babies and Beyond: Moral Considerations," *Homiletic and Pastoral Review* 79 (February 1979): 25–32,

47–49; Rita Arditti, Renata Duelli Klein, and Shelly Minden, eds., *Test Tube Women: What Future for Motherhood* (Boston: Pandora Press, 1984) ◆Gena Corea, *The Mother Machine: Reproductive Technologies from Artificial Insemination to Artificial Wombs* (New York: Harper and Row, 1985).

11. Hall, "Test Tube Babies," 27.

12. Immanuel Jakobovits, "Artificial Insemination," in *Jewish Medical Ethics* (New York: Bloch Publishers, 1975) ◆Fred Rosner, "In Vitro Fertilization and Surrogate Motherhood: The Jewish View," *Journal of Religion and Health* 22 (Summer 1983): 139–60 ◆J. Robert Nelson, "... And Keeps Rebounding/Dilemmas of Conception and Birth," in *Science and Our Troubled Conscience* (Philadelphia: Fortress Press, 1980).

13. Jack Moore, "Human In Vitro Fertilization: Can We Support It?" *Christian Century* 98 (1981): 442–46.

14. George Annas, "Social Policy Implications of Noncoital Reproduction," paper presented at American Society of Law and Medicine, Cambridge, Mass., October 1984.

15. Corea, *Mother Machine.*

16. Charlene Miall, "The Stigma of Involuntary Childlessness," *Social Problems* 33 (April 1986): 268–82.

17. Harris, *"Life* Poll," 52.

Other suggested readings: ◆Lori Andrews, "The Stock Market: The Law of the New Reproduction Technologies," *American Bar Association Journal* 70 (August 1984): 50–56 ◆James M. Childs, Jr., "In Vitro Fertilization: Ethical Aspects and Theological Concerns," *Academy* 36 (1979): 7–20 ◆Herbert Krimmel, "The Case against Surrogate Parenting," *Hastings Center Report* 13 (October 1983): 35–39 ◆Sandra R. Leiblum and Christopher Barbrack, "Artificial Insemination by Donor: A Survey of Attitudes and Knowledge in Medical Students and Infertile Couples," *Journal of Biosocial Science* 15 (1983): 165–72 ◆Fred Rosner and J. D. Bleich, eds., *Jewish Bioethics* (New York: Sanhedrin Press, 1979) ◆Hans O. Tiefel, "Human In Vitro Fertilization: A Conservative View," *Journal of the American Medical Association,* June 18, 1982, 3235–42 ◆John P. Tyler, K. Michael Nicholas, Noel G. Crockett, and Geoffrey Driscoll, "Some Attitudes to Artificial Insemination by Donor," *Clinical Reproduction and Fertility* 2 (1983): 151–60.

Conclusion: An Assessment

1. Russell Baker, *Tinker People, New York Times,* May 24, 1977, 35.

2. Merle J. Berger and Donald P. Goldstein, "Infertility Related to Exposure to DES *in utero:* Reproductive Problems in the Female," in

Miriam D. Mazor and Harriet F. Simons, eds., *Infertility: Medical, Emotional, and Social Considerations* (New York: Human Sciences Press, 1984), 157–68 ◆Alan B. Retik and Stuart B. Bauer, "Infertility Related to DES Exposure *in utero:* Reproductive Problems in the Male," in Mazor and Simons, *Infertility,* 169–79 ◆Daniel Cramer et al., "Tubal Infertility and the Intrauterine Device," *New England Journal of Medicine* 312 (1985): 941.

3. Ruth Hubbard, "The Case against In Vitro Fertilization and Implantation," in Helen Holmes, Betty Hoskins, and Michael Gross, *The Custom-Made Child: Woman-Centered Perspectives* (Englewood Cliffs, N.J.: Humana Press, 1981), 259–60.

4. Shulamith Firestone, *The Dialectic of Sex* (New York: Bantam, 1971).

5. Aldous Huxley, *Brave New World* (New York: Harper and Row, 1979).

6. Gena Corea, *The Mother Machine: Reproductive Technologies from Artificial Insemination to Artificial Wombs* (New York: Harper and Row, 1985).

7. Margaret Atwood, *The Handmaid's Tale* (New York: Houghton Mifflin, 1986) ◆Corea, *Mother Machine.*

8. Meg Dooley, "Helping Mother Nature," *Columbia,* October 1985, 26.

9. Kurt Hirschhorn, "Practical and Ethical Problems in Human Genetics," *Birth Defects* 8 (July 1972): 30.

10. Albert Havercamp and Miriam Orleans, "An Assessment of Electronic Fetal Monitoring," *Women and Health* 7 (1982): 115–34; David Banta, "Benefits and Risks of Electronic Fetal Monitoring," in Helen B. Holmes, Betty B. Hoskins, and Michael Gross, eds., *Birth Control and Controlling Birth* (Clifton, N.J.: Humana Press, 1980), 183–91.

11. Corea, *Mother Machine,* 97.

12. Gail Robinson, "The New Discrimination," *Environmental Action* 10 (March 1979): 4–9; Ronald Bayer, "Women, Work, and Reproductive Hazards," *Hastings Center Report* 12 (October 1982): 14–19 ◆"Four Women Assert Jobs Were Linked to Sterilization," *New York Times,* January 5, 1979, 21.

13. Norma J. Wikler, "Prenatal and Reproductive Technologies: Feminist and Consumer Perspectives," paper presented at American Society of Law and Medicine meetings, Cambridge, Mass., October 1984.

14. Sherry Wieder, Letter to the Editor, *New York Times,* July 9, 1982.

15. Hubbard, "The Case against In Vitro Fertilization and Implantation."

16. Corea, *Mother Machine.*

17. Alexander Morgan Capron, "The New Reproductive Possibilities: Seeking a Moral Basis for Concerted Action in a Pluralistic Society," *Law, Medicine and Health Care,* October 1984 ♦ "Position Paper: Issues Arising from In Vitro Fertilization, Artificial Insemination by Donor, and Related Problems in Biotechnology," *New Zealand Medical Journal* 22 (May 1985): 396–98 ♦ Peter Singer, "Making Laws on Making Babies, *Hastings Center Report,* August 1985, 5–6 ♦ Warnock Committee of Inquiry, "Recommendations," *British Medical Journal,* July 1984, *289.*

18. Personal communication from a director of a sex-selection clinic.

Other suggested readings: ♦ George Annas, "Making Babies without Sex: The Law and the Profits," *American Journal of Public Health,* December 1984, 336–38 ♦ Rita Arditti, Renata Duelli Klein, and Shelly Minden, *Test Tube Women: What Future for Motherhood?* (Boston: Pandora Press, 1984) ♦ Bernard Barber, "In Vitro Fertilization: Public Awareness and Governmental Regulations," *National Forum* 69 (Spring 1979): 32–34 ♦ Sherman Elias and George Annas, "Social Policy Considerations in Noncoital Reproduction," *Journal of the American Medical Association,* January 3, 1986, 62–68 ♦ "Eugenic Artificial Insemination: A Cure for Mediocrity?" *Harvard Law Review* 94 (1981): 1850–70 ♦ Gary Hodgen, "In Vitro Fertilization and Embryo Transfer: Advances in Oocyte Collection," paper presented to American Society of Law and Medicine, Cambridge, Mass., October 1984 ♦ Ruth Hubbard, " 'Fetal Rights' and the New Eugenics," *Science for the People* 16 (March/April 1984): 7–9, 27–29 ♦ R. C. Lewontin, "What Ever Happened to Eugenics?" *Gene WATCH,* Committee for Responsible Genetics 2 (January–April 1985): 8–10 ♦ Ruth Macklin, "Moral Issues in Human Genetics: Counseling or Control?" *Dialogue* 16 (September 1977): 375–96 ♦ Barbara Katz Rothman, "How Science Is Redefining Parenthood," *Ms.,* August 1982, 154–58 ♦ idem, *The Tentative Pregnancy: Prenatal Diagnosis and the Future of Motherhood* (New York: Viking, 1986) ♦ Ann Snitow, "The Paradox of Birth Technology: Exploring the Good, the Bad, and the Scary," *Ms.,* December 1986, 42–46, 76–77 ♦ Nancy Wexler, " 'Will the Circle Be Unbroken?' Sterilizing the Genetically Impaired," in Aubrey Milunsky and George J. Annas, eds., *Genetics and the Law II* (New York: Plenum Press, 1979).

Index